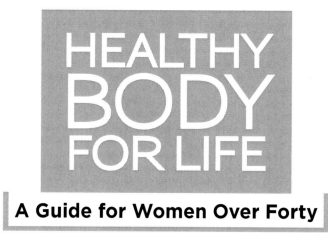

HEALTHY BODY FOR LIFE

A Guide for Women Over Forty

CARLA HAMPSHIRE

You should not undertake any diet/exercise regimen recommended in this book before consulting your personal physician. Neither the author nor the publisher shall be responsible or liable for any loss or damage allegedly arising as a consequence of your use or application of any information or suggestions contained in this book.

ISBN: 978-1-4834-5559-4 (sc)
ISBN: 978-1-4834-5560-0 (hc)
ISBN: 978-1-4834-5561-7 (e)

Library of Congress Control Number: 2016912064

Because of the dynamic nature of the Internet, any web addresses or links contained in this book may have changed since publication and may no longer be valid. The views expressed in this work are solely those of the author and do not necessarily reflect the views of the publisher, and the publisher hereby disclaims any responsibility for them.

Lulu Publishing Services rev. date: 8/19/2016

In loving memory of my mother, Laura, who always guided me with love and wisdom, and who taught me the importance of kindness.

ACKNOWLEDGEMENTS

I wish to thank all the wellness and fitness professionals, friends, and clients for contributing their knowledge, special insights, and personal stories, which helped make this book something I am proud to share with you.

A special thank-you to my husband, Dale, for always supporting my dreams and for being by my side for the past 35 years.

CONTENTS

INTRODUCTION

Live Your Best Life

> " In the end, it's not the years in your life
> that count. It's the life in your years. "
> —Abraham Lincoln

Welcome to *Healthy Body for Life*. The purpose of this guide is to educate and encourage women over 40 to live healthier, happier lives. This is a wonderful time of life. However, it can be filled with many physical and emotional changes, as well as potential health concerns. Despite the challenges you may face, I encourage you to take steps to enhance your wellness.

In *Healthy Body for Life,* you will learn essential principles of health and wellness that will dramatically improve your physical and emotional well-being.

Discover:

- How to remain optimistic about the years to come
- Effective ways to prepare yourself for wellness
- How to meet the nutritional needs for women over 40
- How to stay fit, including an illustrated body-weight workout and a stretching routine
- Strategies to help you cope with hormonal changes

- Tips to help you achieve restorative and rejuvenating sleep
- Simple techniques to reduce the stress in your life

You will also read personal accounts from women just like you and me, who have overcome challenges associated with aging.

I suggest you read *Healthy Body for Life* all the way through to gather the tools and motivation you will need in order to make important lifestyle changes. Then you should keep it as a resource that you can return to time and again.

I invite you to join me on this journey as we explore the pathway to wellness for women over 40. May you find the inspiration to live your best life within the pages of this book.

CHAPTER 1

A Healthy Outlook on Aging

In many cultures around the world, aging is seen as a time of wisdom, grace and continued contribution to society. Elders are still an integral part of their extended families, where they are valued and respected. This makes all the difference to both their mental and physical health. Unfortunately, we sometimes see the opposite in our society. Older people are often regarded as slow, sick, forgetful and of little worth. As soon as it is deemed necessary, they are moved to a retirement home, where they are seldom visited. A rapid decline in their physical and mental health often follows.

How Our Society Defines Aging

> " You can't help getting older, but
> you don't have to get old. "
> —George Burns

This is how our society defines aging.

- Decline in health and wellness
- Decreased freedom and independence
- Lack of contribution to society
- Loss of energy and vitality
- Loss of physical beauty

- Mental and physical decline
- Little value; not mattering anymore

This definition of aging makes us afraid of getting older. Do you believe this to be true for you? Have you accepted that it is all downhill from here? These negative beliefs do not have to become your reality.

No matter how society defines aging, you have to redefine it for yourself. If you accept that there will be a decline in your well-being, then there will be. You have to decide that you will take better care of yourself both physically and mentally. Then you can move forward with a positive outlook and enjoy all the benefits and rewards that come with age: increased confidence, courage, inner strength, freedom, value, knowledge, experience, contribution and love.

I hope that you will draw inspiration from the following three accounts of women in their 40s, 50s and well beyond. The first story is my own. Enjoy!

Courage to Be

> " People grow through experience if they
> meet life honestly and courageously.
> This is how character is built. "
> —Eleanor Roosevelt

When I first started working out in my late 30s, I immediately fell in love with bodybuilding. Upon seeing my interest for the sport, my trainer encouraged me to read all I could about nutrition and bodybuilding. I went to the library and borrowed all the books and magazines I could find on these topics. This is how my journey into health, nutrition and fitness began.

As my knowledge grew, so did my strength and my desire to compete as a bodybuilder. But I told myself that I was too old to be a competitive athlete. This was my story for over nine years—nine years! I had accepted that bodybuilding was a sport for much younger women, and that I, a

2

46-year-old mother of six and a grandmother, had no right to even think about becoming a competitor.

One day, a young trainer who was preparing for an upcoming bodybuilding competition offered to show me the ropes. He would teach me how athletes train and eat as they get ready for competition day. Over the next few weeks, I committed myself to following the stringent diet and dedicated myself to the training. This was the perfect arrangement. I would get to experience what a competitive bodybuilder goes through without having to step on stage. Remember, I still thought I was too old for that. He monitored my progress and encouraged me daily.

The changes I began to see in my physique forced me to re-examine my assumptions. Maybe I wasn't too old. Maybe I could do this. Maybe I had something to offer that might inspire other women my age.

> " Miracles start to happen when you give as much
> energy to your dreams as you do to your fears. "
> —Richard Wilkins

Never underestimate the power of a determined 40-something woman. The love I had for this sport gave me the courage to leap in with both feet. Twelve weeks later, with my husband and children in the audience, I stepped out onto a bodybuilding stage for the very first time to shouts of "Go, Mom!" This exhilarating experience gave me a new sense of confidence. I remember telling myself that from here on in, I would never allow the fear of being "too old" hold me back from positive life experiences. I was ready to take on anything.

From the beginning, I chose to build muscle naturally; this means that I did not use any stimulants, fat burners, steroids, or other harmful drugs. Keeping to this standard, I avoided harming my body with unhealthy and dangerous chemicals and toxins.

I competed several times the following year, finally placing first overall and earning my professional bodybuilder card. If someone had told me that I would one day be a professional bodybuilder, I would have laughed. Yet there I was, trying to hold back tears as I was presented with a prestigious award that would give me the privilege to compete at an international level.

The highlight of my competitive career took place in my early 50s. In October 2012, I flew to the United States to compete in an international-level competition in New Jersey. I had a great coach who helped me get into the best shape of my life. That night, I achieved the highest honour possible in the sport of professional bodybuilding by taking home the first-place award. Becoming an international bodybuilder was like my birthday and Christmas rolled into one!

Fear had held me back for so many years, but my passion for life, for health and for more growing experiences propelled me forward, past my self-imposed barriers of aging. I had dared to try something new. In so doing, I gained a different perspective on what it meant to be a woman over 40. My experiences gave me a new respect for what was possible and what I could accomplish regardless of how old I was.

With my new outlook and courage, I went back to university to finish my Arts and Science degree. Then, my deep interest in nutrition and fitness, gained through the sport of bodybuilding, led me to return to school once again. This time, I became certified in holistic health and nutrition as well as personal fitness training. I wanted to apply this knowledge to help women, especially women of my age group. I realized that women over 40 had different health concerns and needs that were not being fully addressed. I was invited to write articles for fitness magazines on topics of specific interest to this group of women. This inspired me to write a book which discusses the health issues we might face as women over 40, and the steps we can take to improve our well-being.

I am pleased to present my first book to you, *Healthy Body for Life: A Guide for Women over 40*.

Life is full of opportunities to grow, learn and develop no matter how old you are. Is there something you have always wanted to try? Courses you have wanted to take? Something you have wanted to be? You have unlimited potential. Have the courage to open the door to exciting possibilities and expand your horizons in new and wonderful ways.

> " Aging is not lost youth but a new stage
> of opportunity and strength. "
> —Betty Friedan

Feeling Valued

> " As we get older, we have to engage in
> those things that make us feel valued. "
> —Suzanne Truba

Suzanne Truba is the owner of an upscale women's fashion boutique. In 1968, Suzanne imagined that there had to be something more exciting and fulfilling than her employment as a registered nurse. Risking it all, she set out to enhance the state of fashion for women in Calgary by opening her boutique.

Now, despite being in her 70s, Suzanne still runs the store and remains active in her community. In my interview with her, she shared her thoughts about aging and what keeps her feeling young.

Paraphrasing a quote by Satchel Paige, "If you didn't know how old you were, how old would you be?" I believe that so much of aging is a state of mind. I've met women in their 20s who are old, and women in their 80s who are young. Today, women really want to look young, stay fit and live life. Fortunately, our generation is aging differently than our parents because of healthier lifestyles and medical advances.

As one gets older, it is important to always be thankful for what one has, and not to complain about what one hasn't or what might have been. Embracing aging invites more joy, but there is no one road map or model that fits all. We each have to explore what works for us, what keeps us young.

What keeps me young is working in my women's clothing boutique, exercising and spending time with family and friends. Working in my shop offers me fulfilment and purpose. My clients still seek my opinion when it comes to clothing and image; it boosts my self-worth. Exercise is also key for me to aging younger and happier. Regular walking and tennis are an important part of my life each week. Meaningful relationships with family and friends have been and always will be an integral part of my well-being.

In today's North American society, seniors are sometimes, if not often, viewed as has-beens, uninteresting or not valued for their wisdom and life experiences. Perhaps the media has influenced this attitude, because there is so much focus on younger women. As we get older, we have to engage in those things that support our self-worth, make us feel valued and enable us to remain a viable part of society. I don't even talk about retirement anymore!

We all wish to be appreciated, loved and valued no matter how old we are. Focus on those things in your life that make you feel valued, whether in your home, in the workplace or in your community. Continue to seek to add value. But more important, value yourself. You have loved and cared for others for many years. You have knowledge, experience and love worthy of being shared. Celebrate your value! Concentrate on growing better, not older.

Freedom to Fly

> " You are never too old to set another
> goal or to dream a new dream. "
> —C. S. Lewis

Here is Josie Russell's moving story of getting her dream job later in life—a position usually held by much younger women. She had often thought of becoming a flight attendant, but as a mother of four, she had many family responsibilities that made it impossible for her to pursue this goal. Now that her children were older, she had more time to follow that dream. She took a chance and went in for an interview.

When I got home from my job interview, I cried my eyes out. I was convinced I had failed the interview. It had been 20 years since my last interview. It was my girls who picked me up and said, "Mom, if they don't take you, they are going to miss out on something." It was incredible that the support and encouragement I had given them over the years came back to me. You see, I had always wanted to be a flight attendant. Here I was at 46, and I had just lost the opportunity of getting my dream job. I think I was trying so hard to give the perfect answers that I made things worse.

I wanted this so bad that I called them back to apologize for the horrible interview. I asked for a second chance. A while later, they called me back. I got the job, and I love it!

That's a huge accomplishment later in life. Some women say, "I'm too old." No you're not! I was 46 when I got my job of a lifetime. That was everything to me! You know, age is only a number. You have to put yourself out there. You have to keep striving for your goals and dreams. I'm 56 now. I have great kids and a good husband; we are well financially and I have my dream job.

Recognize, just as Josie did, that this is a new stage in your life. Your family responsibilities have changed. Your work life may be different as well. This new time comes with some added freedoms. For Josie, it was the freedom to pursue a career of which she had always dreamed.

What experiences do you want to have? What things do you wish to accomplish? What goals and dreams do you want to fulfil? Remember, "You are never too old to set another goal or to dream a new dream."

Take a moment right now to write down three things that you have always wanted to do. Now narrow it down to one special goal. Write this goal on an index card. On the bottom of the card, write, "What am I going to do today that will take me one step closer to my dream?" Post this on your refrigerator, your bedroom or your bathroom mirror—a place where you will repeatedly see your goal throughout the day. Find a picture that represents your goal, and place it on or beside the card to help you visualize. Take at least one action step each day that will get you closer to accomplishing your goal.

Moving Forward

In the following chapters, you will find the tools you will need in order to live your best life in your 40s and beyond. As you develop a personal health plan and begin to work on improving yourself, you will start to feel better, look better and perform better in all aspects of your life.

I challenge you to move forward with optimism, maximize your health and happiness, prepare to live life to its fullest and enjoy all the benefits that come from living a vibrant and purposeful life. May this new and wonderful stage of your life be a productive one, an expansive one and a healthy one.

CHAPTER 2

Preparing for Wellness—Detoxification

Before we begin our next chapter on nutrition, I feel it is important to talk about detoxification. There is a lot of buzz surrounding this topic as people are becoming more health conscious. However, detoxification is not a new thing. It has been practiced by various cultures and religions around the world for centuries.

What Is Detoxification?

" By cleansing your body on a regular basis and eliminating as many toxins as possible from your environment, your body can begin to heal itself, prevent disease, and become stronger and more resilient than you ever dreamed possible! "
—Dr. Edward Group III

Detoxification is a way of cleansing your body from unhealthy and harmful foods and drinks, medications, environmental pollutants and other irritants. You engage your body's natural ability to process and excrete toxic waste while also reducing the amount of incoming contaminants. During this process, you free your body of accumulated toxins and thereby disease.

Your liver plays a critical role in processing toxins. As the blood passes through your liver, enzymes inactivate and break down toxins so that they can be more readily excreted. Your body excretes toxins in four different ways: through your colon (bowel movements), kidneys (urine), skin (sweat) and lungs (exhaling).

We live in an increasingly toxic world. Our environment and our food and water are not as pure as they were in our grandparents' time. Toxins affect us all, and they are a side effect of living in the modern world.

To help you further understand how toxins can affect you, think of your body as a glass full of water. You can add a few grains of sand (toxins) to this glass of water without affecting the water level too much. What happens when you keep adding sand to your glass without having a way of eliminating the sand that was previously there? The body works the same way. The more toxins accumulate without having a way of cleansing them out, the more your body becomes overloaded and unable to function optimally. This build-up can contribute to the development of degenerative and chronic diseases.

Signs of Toxins in Your Body

" When our bodies become 'toxic', it means that our natural means of ushering out metabolic waste from normal human metabolism, environmental pollution, and what has become known as the Standard American Diet (or SAD diet) have exceeded the threshold for what the body's innate detoxification system can tolerate on its own. With this toxic load, every system in the human body can become affected. From our head to our toes and everything in between, toxicity makes us sick! "
—Dr. Mark Hyman

We acquire toxins in three ways: through physical contact, by ingesting them or by breathing them in. Pollution, chemical irritants, toxic food and impure water are wreaking havoc on our health. Thankfully, the human body has the ability to communicate with us when things are not quite as they should be. It is up to us to pay attention to these messages and take action.

Look at the following list and ask yourself, "Do I suffer from one or more of these symptoms? Is this something that has affected me for a while?" Though we all react differently to toxins, these are some of the common symptoms that can be associated with toxic overload.

- Cognitive problems: brain fog, memory problems
- Depression
- Digestive problems: constipation, bloating, diarrhea, vomiting
- Fatigue
- Inability to lose excess weight
- Neurological issues: balance problems, tremors
- Respiratory congestion: sneezing, coughing, runny nose
- Skin problems: acne, eczema, rashes
- Trouble sleeping
- Unexplained headaches

Note that these symptoms could be more than a result of excess toxins in your body. They may also indicate a medical condition. Consult your doctor about your symptoms.

Toxins can also exacerbate these existing conditions.

- Allergies
- Asthma
- Auto-immune diseases (e.g., lupus, multiple sclerosis, and rheumatoid arthritis)
- Diabetes
- Fibromyalgia

How do you begin to eliminate things that are causing an unnecessary burden on your body? We will look at helpful hints to reduce toxins from your environment and from your food supply. Putting these tips into practice will significantly decrease the strain that toxins place on your body, and they will dramatically improve your health and well-being.

Ways to Reduce Environmental Toxins

There are so many chemicals in our environment, and we cannot possibly avoid them all. They are in our carpets, paint, household cleaners, perfumes and much more. Here are some ways to minimize your exposure to harmful irritants.

- Avoid dry-cleaning your clothes.
- Avoid storing and cooking your food or water in plastic containers. Choose glass, porcelain, or stainless steel containers instead.
- Don't smoke, and avoid being around second-hand smoke.
- Invest in a water filtration system.
- Keep plants in your home that help clean the air and remove toxins, such as the spider plant and the aloe vera plant.
- Minimize your use of the microwave oven.
- Switch to natural, fragrance-free beauty products.
- Use natural household cleaning products and detergents to minimize your exposure to harsh chemicals.

After reading this list, I invite you to commit to making at least one change today. Perhaps instead of using plastic food containers, you can reuse your glass jars to store your leftovers, your bulk items, your spices, or your grab-and-go meal.

Kitchen Cleanse

If you wish to reduce your toxic load, here is a list of some of the food items that should not be in your pantry, refrigerator or freezer. Eliminating or reducing these is a good place to start.

Decide to make at least one change starting today. For example, you may choose to make your own soups from scratch, to avoid the high sodium content of canned soups.

- **Added salt:** Look for the word sodium on the ingredient list. Here are some foods that tend to be high in sodium: soy sauce, salty snacks, canned soups, canned vegetables, frozen meals and smoked or cured foods.

- **Artificial flavours or colours:** Avoid foods with those words on the ingredient list.

- **Artificial sweeteners:** Avoid foods with artificial sweeteners such as aspartame, sucralose, acesulfame potassium and saccharin.

- **Canned foods:** Limit the use of canned foods. Bisphenol-A (BPA) is an industrial chemical used to line food and beverage cans. BPA can seep into your food and beverages.

- **Genetically modified organisms (GMOs):** Some of the most highly genetically modified foods are canola oil, cotton seed oil, corn, soy and sugar from genetically modified sugar beets. If the ingredient list states *sugar*, it is most likely a product sweetened with genetically modified sugar beets. Look for *cane sugar* on the ingredient list instead.

- **High fructose corn syrup:** This is a liquid sweetener made from corn starch. In Canada it is usually labelled as *glucose-fructose* on the ingredient list. It is found in most foods with added sugar and is a common ingredient in processed foods: soft drinks, breakfast cereals, flavoured yogurt, ketchup, canned fruit, jams and baked goods.

- **Monosodium glutamate (MSG):** This food additive and flavour enhancer may appear under different names: yeast extract, auto-lyzed yeast, glutamic acid, natural flavours, hydrolyzed protein and soy protein, to name but a few. It is usually found in processed foods such as gravies, salad dressings, salty snacks, canned soups, frozen dinners and many restaurant foods.

- **Non-organic dairy:** Contains synthetic growth hormone rBGH. Choose organic dairy products instead.

- **Preservatives and additives:** Avoid foods that have a long list of preservatives and additives. These ingredients are usually unpronounceable—for example, butylated hydroxytoluene (BHT), which is used to preserve the freshness of breakfast cereals.

- **Processed foods:** These are convenience foods that are boxed or bagged and come with a long list of ingredients. They are formulated to deliver fat, salt, sugar and chemicals. Choose to cook or bake from scratch with fresh ingredients instead.

- **Sodium nitrate/nitrite:** This is a preservative found in processed meats such as deli meats, bacon and hot dogs. Deli meats containing cultured celery extract and labelled as "natural" are also high in nitrates and nitrites.

- **Trans fats:** Avoid any food with *hydrogenated* or *partially hydrogenated* on the list of ingredients. For example: margarine, shortening, baked goods, cookies, chips and fried foods.

- **Pesticides:** Reduce your intake of pesticides by purchasing organic fruits and vegetables. Consult the Environmental Working Group website (ewg.org) to find a list of produce called the "clean fifteen and the dirty dozen" (Shopper's Guide to Pesticides in Produce). Every year they produce a list of 15 foods that are okay to eat in their conventional state (clean 15) and 12 foods you should only eat organic (dirty dozen).

For the year 2015, out of the 48 fruit and vegetable categories tested, the following 12 fruits and vegetables contained the highest pesticide load, making it safer to purchase these foods organic or grow them yourself.

The Dirty Dozen

Apples	Peaches
Celery	Potatoes
Cherry tomatoes	Snap peas
Cucumbers	Spinach
Grapes	Strawberries
Nectarines	Sweet bell peppers

In 2015, a special addition was made to this list for: kale, collard greens, and hot peppers.

The following 15 fruits and vegetables (the clean 15), were found to have the lowest pesticide load, making them the safest to eat among conventionally grown produce.

The Clean Fifteen

Asparagus	Eggplant	Papayas
Avocados	Grapefruit	Peas (frozen)
Cabbage	Kiwi	Pineapples
Cantaloupe	Mangoes	Sweet corn
Cauliflower	Onions	Sweet potatoes

A small amount of sweet corn and papaya sold in the United States is produced from genetically-engineered (GE) seed stock. Buy organic varieties of these crops if you want to avoid GE produce.

With this list of fruits and vegetables in hand, take a moment now to circle the ones that you purchase on a regular basis. How many of them are from the dirty dozen? How many are from the clean fifteen? On your next shopping trip, commit to making a small change. For example, if you typically purchase conventionally grown apples, try the organic variety instead. By doing this each time you shop, you will slowly convert from dirty to clean.

Cleaning Your Fruits and Vegetables

Whether you are purchasing organic produce or conventionally grown produce, it is a good idea to wash all fruits and vegetables before consuming them. This will help reduce the amount of pesticide residue, bacteria and other germs from your produce. Here is a simple, natural solution you can use to clean your produce.

- Prepare a solution using 3 parts water to 1 part vinegar; place it in a spray bottle
- Spray your fruits and vegetables with this solution
- Let sit for 5 minutes
- Rinse thoroughly with water for 30 seconds

or

- Fill a bowl with 10 parts water to 1 part vinegar
- Soak your fruits and vegetables for 5 minutes, stirring occasionally and rubbing well where appropriate
- Rinse thoroughly with water for 30 seconds

Congratulations—you have taken the first step towards detoxification by simply putting less toxic substances into your body. You have learned how to reduce your exposure to environmental toxins, as well as how to eliminate toxic food from your diet. Now let's look at what you should include in your diet in order to help your body eliminate toxins.

Cleansing Foods

" A healthy outside starts from the inside. "
—Robert Urich

Water

One of the simplest ways to help your body cleanse itself is to drink plenty of purified water. It hydrates the organs so that they can function optimally, it flushes toxins out of the organs and it helps transport that waste out of your body. Our bodies are made up of about 60 percent water, so it makes sense to drink lots of water to stay healthy. The general advice is that we should drink at least eight glasses of water a day.

Lemon Water

Drinking lemon water serves to stimulate the liver's purification process. First thing in the morning, add the juice of one-quarter to one-half a lemon to a glass of warm water. Its bitterness helps encourage a bowel movement. It is also a natural diuretic that increases the flow of urine to help flush out toxins. Remember to rinse your mouth after drinking lemon water, to protect your tooth enamel.

Eat Your Greens

Dark leafy greens are bursting with nutrients and disease-fighting antioxidants. They are naturally low in calories and high in fibre. This acts as a scrub brush for your digestive tract, detoxifying as it passes through to the colon. As an alkaline food, it also helps to soothe inflammation in your body. Include these excellent leafy greens in your diet: arugula, beet greens, bok choi, broccoli, cabbage, collard greens, dandelion, kale, mustard greens, romaine lettuce, spinach, swiss chard and turnip greens.

Drink Your Greens

Raw, freshly made vegetable and fruit juices are rich in vitamins, minerals, enzymes and trace elements. These are beneficial to your health and help prevent disease. In juice form, these nutrients are easily assimilated without putting a strain on your digestive organs. Besides being highly nourishing, fresh juices also help your body to detoxify. As alkaline juices nourish your cells, they begin to release acids (toxins) that can then be removed through the elimination channels. You will learn more about juicing later on in this chapter.

Berries

Just like greens, berries are packed with antioxidants and are high in fibre. This cleansing and nourishing food aids your body's natural detoxification process. Fresh blueberries, raspberries, blackberries and strawberries are excellent choices.

Dandelion Tea

One cup of roasted dandelion root tea taken at bedtime will help stimulate your liver to release toxins. As a diuretic, it will increase detoxification through urination. Check with your doctor before taking this tea because it may interact with some medications.

Chlorella

Chlorella is a single-celled, freshwater micro-algae, widely used as a supplement among the Japanese and prized as a superfood. It is rich in chlorophyll, which is a powerful detoxifier. Chlorella has the unique ability to bind to metals and chemicals and usher them out of the body. It is available at your local health food store in powder, capsules and tablets.

Spirulina

Spirulina is chlorella's older cousin; its use dates back to the ninth century. It is a microscopic blue-green, freshwater algae. Just like chlorella, spirulina is rich in chlorophyll, making it a powerful detoxifier. It also has a unique combination of phytonutrients (plant nutrients), which can help cleanse the body from the onslaught of toxins it is exposed to on a daily basis. It is available at your local health food store in powder, capsules and tablets.

I encourage you to review this list and decide which foods you will include in your daily diet. For example, including more greens and berries will not only increase your overall nutrition, but it will also help keep your body cleansed from toxins to which you may be exposed.

Five Ways to Cleanse through Your Skin

The skin is your body's largest organ of elimination. Up to one-third of toxins are eliminated through your skin. Here are five easy ways to help promote detoxification through your skin.

1. Dry Skin Brushing

Dry skin brushing is a simple, daily treatment that gets rid of dead skin cells and unclogs your pores, opening up the channels of elimination through your skin. As an added bonus, it improves blood and lymph circulation, helping the liver and lymph nodes deal with unwanted, harmful materials.

Begin by purchasing a long-handled brush with natural bristles. Prior to your morning shower:

- Stand in the tub and brush your entire body with firm yet gentle strokes, beginning at your feet and moving up the legs, stomach, chest, arms, and back. Avoid sensitive areas such your breasts and your face. Brush each area several times, and always brush upwards towards your neck; this is the direction in which the lymph flows.
- Brush for two to five minutes.
- Follow with a hot shower. Gradually turn to cold water to stimulate circulation.

Remember to clean your brush once a week with soap and water, and leave it to air dry.

2. Cleanse with a Sugar Scrub

Gently scrubbing the skin with a natural product has beneficial effects similar to those of dry skin brushing. Sugar scrubs exfoliate and detoxify your skin, revealing healthier, glowing skin without the use of harsh chemicals.

Here is a basic sugar scrub recipe that can be made with ingredients from your kitchen. Mix the following ingredients together and store them in a glass jar with a tight fitting lid until ready to use.

- 1 cup coconut palm sugar or brown sugar
- 1/2 cup olive oil or almond oil
- A few drops of pure vanilla extract (optional)

On your wet skin, rub a handful of this mixture in circular motions all over your body, beginning with your feet and moving your way upwards. Be gentle with the more sensitive skin of your face. Please use caution because the tub may become slippery.

3. Use the Steam Room or Sauna

Looking back through history, even ancient civilizations knew the many benefits of using heat and steam therapies. They bathed in public steam baths or natural hot springs to improve health, relaxation and beauty.

The heat and steam open up your skin's pores and allow this healing moisture to reach deep into your dermis to help cleanse and detoxify. Through perspiration, your body is better able to release toxins. Sweat helps transport impurities such as unhealthy minerals, chemicals and heavy metals to your skin's surface, where they are released. Dead skin cells are also flushed out, leaving you with a healthier glow. It is important to cleanse your skin with a nice, cool shower after your steam bath; this removes the toxins and dead skin cells that have been discharged. It also helps to close the enlarged pores and improves your circulation.

Spend anywhere between 10–20 minutes in a steam room one to three times per week. Steam rooms can be found in most health clubs, gyms or community centres.

Steam baths may not be recommended for those suffering from high blood pressure, a heart condition or diabetes. Check with your doctor.

4. Enjoy an Epsom Salts Bath

If you cannot get to a steam room, an Epsom salts bath is a great alternative. It will help with the detoxification process, encourages relaxation and will significantly reduce overall tension and muscle aches.

Fill a bathtub with water as hot as is comfortable. Add one to two cups of Epsom salts crystals to the bath water and allow this to dissolve. This produces a great mineral treatment to help remove toxins from your body. To enhance the relaxation effect, you may add six to eight drops of your favourite essential oils to the bath water; lavender is a good choice. A 20-minute bath one to three times a week can be a great addition to your health and wellness regimen.

Epsom salts baths may not be recommended for those suffering from high blood pressure, a heart condition or diabetes. Check with your doctor.

5. Use an Air-dried Towel

After your bath or shower, dry your skin with a towel that has been air-dried. The roughness of the fabric will help scrub off dead skin cells and improve your circulation. Do this once a week.

Detox by Losing Body Fat

Your body naturally eliminates toxins on a regular basis through its elimination channels: the urinary tract, the colon, the skin, and the lungs. What happens when your body is overloaded with toxins, when the incoming toxins exceed the rate at which you can eliminate them? When we eat in excess of what our body needs, the extra calories are stored as body fat. The same thing happens with excess toxins. Your body protects itself by getting them out of circulation and away from vital organs, storing them in your fatty tissue.

If you are overweight, you probably have an accumulation of toxins. By losing body fat through a detoxification protocol, you not only lose weight but will also release toxins from your fat cells. Therefore losing weight and maintaining a healthy weight is important to keeping your body free of toxins.

Losing body fat requires more than just detoxification. Proper nutrition and exercise will further assist you in your quest to reduce unhealthy body fat. You will learn more about the importance of food and exercise in the next two chapters.

Detox with Yoga

A yoga practice which stretches, compresses and twists every part of your body will help with the removal of waste products that build up in your body. Yoga twists are especially effective in stimulating digestion and elimination by squeezing the abdominal organs. Let's learn a basic pose, the seated twist (Marichyasana III).

Seated Twist (Marichyasana III)

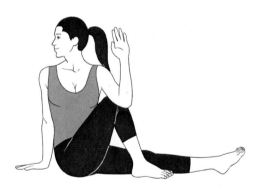

- Sit tall on a mat. Bend the right leg and place the right foot flat on the mat.
- Rest your right hand on the floor behind you for support.
- Rotate your torso to the right, and bring your left elbow to the outside of your right knee.
- Exhale as you gently press your left elbow into your right knee to encourage your torso to twist.

- Inhale and twist a little more with each exhalation for five deep breaths.
- Release and then repeat on the other side for five deep breaths.

Take a moment right now to try the seated twist.

Holly Blazina, a rehabilitative yoga instructor, explains how yoga, and especially the yoga twists, helped her overcome chronic fatigue.

> I struggled with chronic fatigue when I was younger. My organs were depleted. One of the things that helped me come out of that was yoga. I believe that one of the reasons why is because of the effect it had on my organs.
>
> By doing yoga twists, there is a squeezing and soaking effect on the organs. It's like squeezing a sponge. You are squeezing out the toxins, and as the organs expand again, new circulation is brought in. Just like when you have a dirty sponge, and you put it in water, then squeeze it out and allow it to expand. If you keep repeating this process, eventually a lot of the junk is going to come out of that sponge.

Look for a yoga class in your neighbourhood to help keep you at your best inside and out.

Ten Health Benefits of Reducing Your Toxic Load

Reducing your toxic load can lead to many health benefits, including:

- A greater sense of well-being
- A sharper mind
- Better digestion
- Clearer skin
- Feeling lighter
- Improved immune function

- More energy
- Reduced cravings
- Reduced stress
- Reduced weight

Reducing toxins can also be a great springboard to healthier habits. Once you experience the health benefits that come from freeing yourself of toxins, you will be less likely to return to your old ways. It will help you ease into making lifestyle changes that will continue to promote health and well-being.

Juicing for Health

" Since juicing, I have regained my vitality. "
—Sue Hetherington

I interviewed David W. Rowland, Professor Emeritus (Edison Institute of Nutrition) and author of many health publications, including *The Vitamost Encyclopedia of Food Based Medicines*. He stressed that sometimes we make detoxification a lot more complicated than it needs to be. These are some of his thoughts on the subject.

> Detoxification is great! You can't nourish yourself if you're getting strangled in your own waste products. The easiest way to detoxify the body is to stop putting the garbage in. The body has its own eliminative processes. For example, you can be exposed to moderate amounts of heavy metals. If your body is nourished well, it can get rid of them all by itself.

> However, if you are not nourished well, and you are overstressed, and you are overexposed to heavy metals, then you may need to take specific therapy for that. But, I repeat, if you just stop putting the garbage in, it gives your body a chance to catch up with the overload.

Unfortunately for some people, elimination is not enough. You may need a few days of vegetable juices to give your system a break in order to catch up.

The following story is Sue Hetherington's personal detox experience. She is a support worker who provides one-on-one help for the elderly. Sue hadn't been feeling well for quite some time. She realized that if she wanted to continue in this line of work, she had to take better care of herself. She knew that she had some lifestyle habits to change.

> I was living with constant pain in my liver area. I loved having two glasses of wine as I cooked dinner every night, and a third glass with dinner. But in September of last year, I stopped drinking alcohol. I decided that I did not want to follow down the same road my father did. He passed away at the exact age I am now, 54, from alcoholism.

> I contacted my doctor, and he wanted to put me on pills. I said no! I decided to go about it alternatively. I did some research on detoxification and watched the movie featuring Joe Cross, *Fat, Sick and Nearly Dead*. I think every person should watch it.

> I took what I learned to my naturopathic doctor and told her that I wanted to do a 10-day juice detox. This means drinking only freshly juiced vegetables and fruits for a 10-day period. She was wholeheartedly on board and gave me a supplement to support my liver. I wanted to rebuild my liver; I wanted it strong. I truly believe in my heart that most of the illnesses we suffer from these days are due to an overstressed, overworked, fatty and malnourished liver. The liver filters everything!

> I am sure that everything I was filtering was coming right back in. It was a revolving cycle. I was getting the flu and

colds, and headaches and migraines would have me in bed for a couple of days. I felt very drawn, very tired and completely worn out. In addition, I was diagnosed with glaucoma about a year ago. This was something that weighed heavily on my mind. That's why I decided to do a 10-day juice detox.

I concocted my own recipes. I wanted every single juice to have leafy greens like kale or spinach. I also added cucumber, carrots, beets, and apples and oranges for the extra vitamin C. First thing in the morning, I would have hot lemon water with a piece of ginger; lemon is good for flushing. Then I would sip on 16–20 ounces of freshly made juice. Then for my midmorning snack, I would have 8–10 ounces of juice. My lunch consisted of another 20 ounces. In the mid-afternoon, I would drink ginger tea. And for my dinner, I would have another 20 ounces. This takes a lot of vegetables, but for me, it was worth it!

I'm never going to look back because it was an amazing journey. I feel so much better. I don't get headaches anymore. My mind, my skin and my eyes are clearer. I don't require glasses all day now, which is quite remarkable. My spirituality has come back, and the liver pain is gone! I didn't do this to lose weight, but I did lose 14 pounds, and I lost my cravings too.

Since juicing, I also found that I have regained my vitality. I used to be a bodybuilder and worked out all the time. But as of late, I have been having trouble going up the stairs without breathing hard. Since the detox, my husband and I go for five-mile walks, and we walk hard! I feel so much better. I can breathe deeply without stressing or straining. My goal is to build my strength back up to where I can run again.

I spoke with Sue again a few months after our initial interview. She reported that since speaking with me, she has made some important changes in her professional life. Feel her enthusiasm as she tells of her new-found direction.

> My interview with you made me take stock of what I really wanted to do with my life. It was pivotal in my changing direction. I have since left my position in health care as a support worker. I am now going to dedicate my life as a health and wellness advocate. I have never felt as positive, in tune and happy with my life as I do now. Thank you!

Weekend Detox

There are many detox protocols available. You can find them online, in books or from a healthcare professional. If this is your first time cleansing, or if you have a high toxic load, you should only do a detox with supervision from a holistic nutritionist or naturopathic doctor.

A gradual approach to detoxification is always recommended. This prevents a sudden release of large amounts of toxins into the bloodstream. Your body cannot process a high amount of toxins at once; these will likely reabsorb and cause problems such as headaches, fatigue and skin issues.

Here is a mini fruit and vegetable juice cleanse anyone can do over a weekend. This is a great way to give your body a break so that it can catch up on its detoxification and elimination processes. This is also an excellent way to begin a weight loss program. Anything longer than this should be done with the guidance of a healthcare professional.

Choose a weekend where you don't have much planned. A long weekend is preferable.

Friday should be a day where you lighten the amount of food you take in. This will help prepare you for a two-day juice fast.

- On Friday morning, drink a glass of warm water with the juice of half an organic lemon. This helps to stimulate the digestive tract.
- Eat only vegetables and fruit on this day, with a focus on the vegetables. These can be raw or steamed. Organic produce is preferred, because you do not wish to add to your toxic load.
- Drink at least eight glasses of water a day, preferably more, during this cleanse period.

What to Include in Your Juices

On Saturday morning, you will begin juicing vegetables and fruit for your meals and snacks for the next two days. These juices are packed with nutrients that will help sustain you. The large amount of soluble fibre will help with detoxification and elimination.

You will require about 72 ounces (just over 2 litres) of juice per day: 16 ounces (2 cups, or about 500 mL) each for breakfast, lunch and dinner, and 8 ounces (1 cup, or about 250 mL) each for your between-meal snacks, and for after dinner if you are hungry.

Pour the juice into glass containers, seal tightly and store in the refrigerator. All juices should include:

- Leafy greens (kale, spinach, swiss chard, collard greens, romaine lettuce)
- A watery vegetable (cucumber, celery)
- A sweet vegetable (carrots, beets)
- Fruit (apple, pear, pineapple, watermelon)

You may also wish to add ginger root, mint leaves, cilantro or parsley to your juice to aid digestion and improve cleansing. Use these in moderation because they may overpower the taste of your juice.

This will cost about $10 a day in fresh produce, and it will likely take you 30 minutes to wash and prepare the fruits and vegetables, juice them and clean up afterwards.

There are a variety of juicers on the market. The one I use is a juicer by Breville.

If you love experimenting with exciting recipes, then you will want to check out the book by Joe Cross, *The Reboot with Joe Juice Diet*. Here is a juice recipe from Joe's book.

Green Carrot Ginger (Green Juice)—makes about 16 ounces (enough for one meal)

Ingredients:

- 2 cucumbers
- 8 carrots
- 6 kale leaves
- 1 pear
- 2-inch (5 cm) piece of fresh ginger root

For Saturday and Sunday, follow the meal schedule outlined below.

- In the morning, drink a glass of warm water with the juice of half an organic lemon.
- Breakfast: drink 16 ounces of juice.
- Mid-morning snack: drink 8 ounces of juice.
- Lunch: drink 16 ounces of juice.
- Mid-afternoon snack: drink 8 ounces of juice.
- Dinner: drink 16 ounces of juice.
- After-dinner snack: drink 8 ounces of juice.

Drink extra water and tea such as dandelion root or ginger tea in between meals to help with the detoxification process.

Juicing versus Smoothies

People often ask, "What is the difference between juicing and making a smoothie?" They are both excellent ways of adding more fruits and vegetables to your daily diet.

Juicing is ideal when detoxifying. You use a juicer to extract the juice from fruits and vegetables. It provides your body with all the vitamins, minerals and phytonutrients it needs while being very light on the digestive system.

A smoothie is a denser beverage made in a blender from fruits, vegetables, added juice or milk. It can be used as a meal replacement or a snack.

Additional Tips to Help You Get the Most out of This Weekend Cleanse

- Enjoy an Epsom salts bath every night before bed. This will help you relax and also help you release toxins.
- Make an appointment with your massage therapist. This too will help with relaxation and toxin release.
- Take time to do some gentle yoga or stretching.
- Go for walks.
- Listen to quiet music.
- Take time to meditate.
- Read a good book.
- Turn off distractions such as the television.
- Enjoy a nap in the afternoon.

After this weekend cleanse, you will feel lighter and have increased energy and mental focus. I encourage you to check your calendar and choose a detox weekend now. Look at it as a spa weekend for yourself.

Moving Forward after a Cleanse

After a cleanse, you will feel so well that you may not want to rush back to your regular diet. As a matter of fact, you should ease back into eating. The day after your weekend cleanse, I recommend you eat fruit and lightly steamed vegetables along with eggs, beans and lentils. The following day, if you wish to return to eating meat, do so slowly, eating only one portion of organic chicken.

Moving forward, you will also benefit from eating more lightly than you were prior to your cleanse. Doing so will lighten the load on your digestive system and prevent a build-up of toxins. Eat slowly and enjoy your food; avoid eating until you are completely full. This is a good rule to live by, to prevent overeating and overburdening your system.

CHAPTER 3

Nutrition for Women Over 40

❝ Let food be thy medicine and medicine be thy food. ❞
—Hippocrates

Nutrition plays a very important role at this stage of your life; it is the key to vitality and good health as you age. Eating the right food will help keep your hormones balanced, keep your weight under control, improve your bone health, keep your heart and mind healthy and help your digestive system function optimally. But before we begin talking about specifics to women over 40, let's review some basics we all learned in Biology 101.

Nutrition Basics

What Are Proteins?

Proteins are organic molecules made up of amino acids, the building blocks of life. Their main function is to build, repair and maintain body tissue such as muscles and organs. Protein foods can come from animal sources (lean red meat, poultry, fish, eggs, dairy), or from vegetarian sources (green leafy vegetables, beans and lentils, grains, nuts and seeds, soy). Protein provides four calories per gram. There are two types of amino acids, essential and non-essential.

Essential amino acids are necessary for healthy growth and maintenance of the body. They cannot be synthesized in the body, and therefore they must be obtained from the diet. Animal-based foods contain all of the essential amino acids. Plant-based foods are also good sources of essential amino acids.

Non-essential amino acids can be synthesized in the body, which means they can be produced from other compounds found in the body.

What Are Carbohydrates?

Carbohydrates are our main source of energy. They are broken down into simple sugars to help fuel us. Carbohydrates provide four calories per gram. There are two types of carbohydrates, simple and complex.

Simple carbohydrates are found in white sugar, honey, soft drinks, processed fruit juice, candy and other sweet snacks, white bread, white rice and boxed cereal. They are processed quickly and give you a brief boost of energy.

Complex carbohydrates are more fibrous foods such as whole grains and their products (oats, brown rice, quinoa, whole grain bread and pasta), green vegetables, starchy vegetables (sweet potatoes, squash, potatoes), and beans and lentils. Their higher fibre content means that they will take more time to process, giving sustained energy over a longer period of time.

To which category does fruit belong? It is digested quickly, giving you a burst of energy much like simple carbohydrates. But it is also rich in fibre, which slows down its digestion. Therefore, fruit is a little bit of both.

What Are Fats?

Fats are an important part of a healthy diet. They are a concentrated source of energy and have many other important roles. Fats help the body dissolve, absorb and store the fat-soluble vitamins A, D, E and K. They also help develop the brain, regulate the production of sex hormones, keep the nervous system in good health, strengthen the immune system, provide cushioning to protect the internal organs and keep the skin and hair healthy.

Fats are a denser food that helps keep us fuller longer, providing nine calories per gram. Some healthy sources of fat are avocados, nuts and seeds and their butters, fatty fish such as salmon and sardines, and oils such as coconut oil, flax seed oil and olive oil. Limit fats that can cause inflammation and disease, such as fats from red meat, full-fat cheese, deep-fried foods and processed foods such as pastries and chips.

Essential fatty acids (**EFAs**) are required for many important biological processes. They are essential to health but cannot be synthesized in the body, and therefore they must be obtained from the foods in our diet.

There are two fatty acids that are essential for humans: omega-3 and omega-6 fatty acids. Our Western diet generally contains enough, if not too much, omega-6 fatty acids in the form of various plant oils and animal products. Too much of this fatty acid can contribute to disease. Focus instead on including more omega-3 foods in your diet. Omega-3 fatty acids have anti-inflammatory properties and protect us from degenerative diseases. They have also been found to help reduce bothersome symptoms of menopause such as hot flashes and mood swings. Some food sources of omega-3 fatty acids are fatty fish such as salmon and sardines, flax seed oil, and nuts and seeds such as almonds, pecans, walnuts, ground flax seeds, chia seeds and pumpkin seeds.

What Is Fibre?

Fibre is the portion of plant foods that our digestive system cannot completely break down. Dietary fibre is found in vegetables and fruits, grains, nuts and seeds, and beans and lentils. Eating fibrous foods is important for digestive health. Fibre acts as a scrub brush for the digestive tract. The amount of fibre women should obtain from their diet is at least 25 grams per day. There are two types of fibre; soluble and insoluble. Both pass through our bodies undigested.

Soluble fibre binds with water to form a gel that helps eliminate waste, reduces blood sugar by slowing glucose absorption and has a cholesterol-lowering effect.

Insoluble fibre remains mostly undigested as it passes through the digestive tract. It helps eliminate waste by adding bulk to the stool.

Both types of fibre help keep our bowel movements regular. Most fibrous foods contain a little of both types of fibre. For example, a large apple contains five grams of dietary fibre in both forms. The pectin in the apple is the soluble fibre, and the skin is the insoluble fibre.

Studies show that our modern diet does not include enough dietary fibre. Despite the recommendation that we increase our daily fibre intake, many of us are afraid that this may cause digestive discomfort and bloating. Here are some practical suggestions on how to increase your intake without experiencing uncomfortable symptoms.

- Increase your fibre intake gradually. Include an additional portion of fibre-rich foods every few days.
- Spread out fibre-rich foods throughout the day instead of consuming them all in the same meal.
- Increase your water intake to at least eight cups a day to help the body utilize fibre more effectively.

Why Do We Need Water?

Water is essential and plays a vital role in many functions. It hydrates all body tissues and helps regulate body temperature. It helps break down food for digestion and assists in the distribution of nutrients and oxygen to the cells throughout the body. It also helps remove waste via urine, bowel movements, sweat and breathing. A good rule of thumb is to drink eight glasses (about two litres) of water a day. Extra water is required if you are exercising or if you are ill. If you want to be more specific, here is a formula to help you know how much water you should drink on a daily basis.

Divide your body weight (in pounds) in half. This is how many ounces of water you should drink in a day. For example, if you weigh 160 pounds (72.5 kg), you should be drinking 80 ounces (about 2.5 litres) of water daily. This amounts to ten 8 ounce (250 mL) glasses of water.

Formulas aside, take a good look at how much water you are drinking now, and strive to improve upon that.

Vitamins and Minerals

Vitamins and minerals are substances that are found in the food we eat. They are necessary for normal growth, development and activity. We cannot make most of these compounds in our bodies, and therefore it is essential that we eat a variety of foods from fresh, clean and healthy sources in order to obtain a wide range of these health-giving substances. Taking a daily multivitamin and multimineral supplement is a good way to enhance the diet, but it should not be a replacement for proper nutrition.

How Food Affects Your Hormone Balance

Lois Garton has been a practitioner of traditional Chinese medicine (TCM) for over 25 years. She explains why nutrition is key to maintaining hormone balance as you age.

> If the body is well balanced going into menopause, any problems encountered are going to be minimized. The hormonal changes are going to be easier for the body to manage. If you have a body that has been out of balance for 20 or 30 years, that will contribute to having more of a problem when the hormones begin to change.

> In Chinese medicine, the kidney energy is the mother of all energy. This energy naturally depletes as we age; our hair turns grey and our skin ages. How do you keep the kidney energy strong? First, don't expend your

energy carelessly. Second, eat well to keep your energy replenished.

In TCM theory, it is the spleen that works to provide the nutritive energy necessary to buoy up the kidney energy. Interestingly, in TCM, the spleen is involved not only in good digestion and absorption of nutritive energy, but also in maintaining a balanced hormonal system. So you really do have to eat well and regularly!

I see women in their 50s who have been pushing themselves every day and following poor dietary habits. When they hit menopause, the wheels fall off. These are the women who are likely to have more severe menopausal symptoms.

Get yourself balanced in your 30s and 40s so that at menopause, if you have problems, they will be less severe and easier to address.

Proper nourishment is a good starting point when it comes to keeping the hormones balanced. Hormonal transitions such as menopause can be supported by a nutrient-dense diet consisting of whole foods. Include quality protein sources, antioxidant-rich fruits and vegetables, and hormone-balancing dietary fats in your daily nutrition.

You Have to Eat Well

Eating food high in nutrients will keep your body functioning optimally and give you a better chance at managing your hormonal changes. As Lois stated, "You have to eat well!"

Protein: As you age, your muscle mass decreases. After age 30, you can lose up to 5 percent of your muscle mass per decade, especially if you are inactive. Since muscle is more metabolically active, meaning that it burns more calories to stay alive, a loss of muscle mass can lead to weight gain.

It can also lead to a loss of strength and function, which can affect your independence. By eating protein foods, you can help maintain most of your muscle mass as you age. Protein also helps to balance the hormones in your body, such as the thyroid hormones, which regulate metabolism.

Protein should be included at every meal and snack, evenly distributed throughout your day. Healthy choices are lean poultry, wild-caught fish, eggs, beans and lentils, nuts and seeds and their butters, protein powder and low-fat dairy. Begin with a breakfast high in protein such as an egg omelette, or a protein smoothie.

Fruits and Vegetables: Eat a variety of colourful fruits and vegetables. If you find it difficult to include adequate amounts of fruits and vegetables in your daily diet, try juicing or including them in smoothies. Berries and dark leafy greens are an excellent choice. These nutritious foods contain high amounts of disease-fighting antioxidants.

Cruciferous vegetables such as broccoli, Brussels sprouts, cabbage and cauliflower contain the phytochemical indole-3-carbinol. This compound can help balance estrogen levels by promoting healthy metabolism of estrogen. It reduces the negative side effects typically associated with excess estrogen. This helps women who are experiencing symptoms of premenstrual syndrome (PMS), as well as perimenopausal and menopausal issues such as hot flashes. This particular group of vegetables is also very beneficial in reducing the risk of breast cancer.

Fats: Fad diets often steer women away from eating dietary fats. However, you need healthy fats every day in order for the hormonal system and nervous system to function well. Excellent sources of healthy fats are avocados, nuts and seeds and their butters, fatty fish such as salmon and sardines, and oils such as coconut oil, flax seed oil and olive oil.

Flax seeds are an important nutrient for supporting healthy estrogen levels because they contain phytoestrogens. This is a nutrient found in plants that may act like estrogen in the body. If you are experiencing estrogen deficiency issues such as decreased libido, urinary incontinence, thinning bones, vaginal dryness, or dry hair and skin, include a tablespoon of ground flax seeds in your salads, oatmeal or smoothies every day.

Foods to Avoid

- Processed foods are mostly devoid of nutrients. They only serve to fill you up and leave less room for the healthier foods you should be eating. But more important, they can disrupt hormone balance.
- Sugary treats and other simple carbohydrates such as white flour can contribute to fatigue, cravings, mood swings, PMS, hot flashes, insomnia and weight gain.
- Alcohol, caffeine, spicy foods and high-fat foods can contribute to the incidence of menopausal symptoms such as hot flashes.

See chapter 5 on hormone management for more food tips.

Weight Management

You are over 40 with an expanding waistline, and your weight keeps rising. You might be wondering, "What's happening to me?" The middle-age spread has become a reality. You eat less and exercise more, yet you are still fighting the battle of the bulge. This affects your appearance, your energy levels, your quality of life and your health. So what is causing this change? It can be a more sedentary lifestyle, a change in your diet, changing hormones, reduced muscle mass, a slower metabolism or a combination of factors.

Let's examine your nutrition. Are you eating too much, or perhaps not enough? Are you always on a diet? Are you eating all the wrong foods?

Eat Enough

We've all heard this simple solution to losing weight: "Eat less, move more!" Unfortunately some women take this to extremes, eating far less than their bodies require to function normally. Have you ever thought of starving yourself to lose weight? Think again. You may actually be setting yourself up for weight gain and derailing your weight-loss efforts.

The energy your body requires comes from two places: fat reserves, or your daily food intake. Drastically decreasing the amount of calories you take in on a daily basis will definitely lead to short-term weight loss. This will make you believe that if you continue depriving yourself of adequate amounts of food, you will eventually reach your ideal weight. Unfortunately, you have now successfully slowed down your metabolism, meaning that you will burn calories at a slower rate. Once you resume eating normally, your body will have a tendency to hold on to calories consumed. If you allow starvation to become a habit, you will actually be contributing to your own weight gain in the future.

Basal Metabolic Rate

Let's talk about your basal metabolic rate. Your BMR is the rate at which your body burns calories while at rest. These calories are used for essential functions such as breathing, digestion and circulation. An approximate formula to find out how many calories your body needs just for survival is as follows: weight in pounds × 10, or weight in kilograms × 22.

For example, if you weigh 160 pounds, the formula would look like this: $160 \times 10 = 1,600$ daily calories. This is your BMR.

After you calculate your BMR, consider your activity level to account for calories burned during exercise, and multiply your BMR by the number below that best reflects this.

- BMR × 1.2 if you are mainly sedentary (little or no exercise)
- BMR × 1.375 if you are performing light exercise (leisurely walking or household chores for 30–50 minutes, 3–4 days per week)
- BMR × 1.55 if you are performing moderate exercise or sports (30–60 minutes, 3–5 days per week)
- BMR × 1.725 if you are an active individual (45–60 minutes, 6–7 days per week at moderate to high intensity)

Here are the calculations done for you. Find your weight and match it to your current activity level to find out how many calories you should be eating on a daily basis to maintain your current weight.

Weight	BMR	Sedentary	Light Exercise	Moderate Exercise	Active
120 lbs / 54 kg	1200	1400	1650	1860	2070
140 lbs / 63 kg	1400	1680	1925	2170	2415
160 lbs / 72 kg	1600	1920	2200	2480	2760
180 lbs / 81 kg	1800	2160	2475	2790	3105
200 lbs / 91 kg	2000	2400	2750	3100	3450
220 lbs / 100 kg	2200	2640	3025	3410	3795

For example, if your BMR indicates 1600 calories, and you walk leisurely for 30 minutes three times a week, this is how many calories you need to consume in order to fuel your activities: $1600 \times 1.375 = 2200$ calories. If you want to maintain this weight, you would continue eating about 2200 calories a day. If you wish to lose weight, you could do it by reducing the number of daily calories, by increasing the number of calories burned through daily activity, or ideally a combination of both.

Don't reduce calories below what your BMR states is necessary for essential bodily functions. In this example, don't go lower than 1600 calories. This would result in a slower metabolism and not in your desired weight loss. As you lose weight, recalculate your BMR.

Don't Diet

Every few years, there seems to be a new fad diet that becomes the craze: high-protein diet, low-carb diet, low-fat diet—the list goes on. The popularity of fad diets is their ability to provide quick weight loss.

Many of these diets do result in weight loss. But diets are not sustainable and are typically not good sources of long-term nutrition. Your body will crave the nutrients that it is missing. It will continue to crave more and more food to satisfy its malnourishment, leading to eventual weight gain. Diets can also cause rebound effects in the form of more weight gain due to a damaged metabolism. You may also become vitamin deficient and develop other health complications.

The problems that can occur when you follow fad diets can range from mild to severe. Mild symptoms include diarrhea, nausea, headaches and moodiness. More severe health complications include vitamin deficiency, heart disease, high blood pressure and high triglycerides. What further complicates the issue is that most people will not know they have a problem until the condition progresses to dangerous levels. This is one of the reasons why any diet modifications should first be discussed with your doctor.

A Healthy Metabolism

Here are eight simple rules to help you develop a healthy metabolism that will assist your weight management goals.

1. Drink adequate water
2. Eat enough for your needs
3. Eat fibrous foods
4. Eat more often (every 3 to 4 hours)
5. Eat protein at every meal
6. Eat smaller meals
7. Never skip breakfast
8. Practice portion control: 1/2 of your plate for vegetables, 1/4 for protein, and 1/4 for starchy carbohydrates

Food Swapping

Processed foods bog down your system, slow down your metabolism and increase your daily caloric intake above what you need for daily living. Start by replacing processed foods with whole foods. For example, eat fruit instead of drinking sugar-laden juice. Use spices in your cooking and salads instead of fatty sauces and dressings. Eat oatmeal instead of sugary cereals. Replace spaghetti with spaghetti squash. Snack on nuts instead of doughnuts.

These whole foods are far higher in vitamins, minerals and dietary fibre, and they are lower in sugar and fat than processed foods. Swapping for healthier foods is a great place to start if you wish to lose weight the healthy way. Trade in your processed foods for a whole-foods diet rich in fruits and vegetables, lean protein, grains, beans and lentils, nuts and seeds, and healthy fats.

Keep Track

Keeping track of what you eat and drink is a great way to help you assess the quantity and quality of the food you are having throughout the day. As you write things down, you become more aware of what you are eating, and this may prevent you from overeating. It keeps you personally accountable and may help you make healthier choices. In addition, recording the time of your meal can help you check if you are eating at regular intervals. You may also wish to record the mood you were in while eating (stressed, in a hurry, sad, etc.).

Here is an example of a chart you can use. There are also many phone apps that help you track your food. Use what works best for you.

Meals & Snacks	e.g., 2 slices whole wheat bread with 1 tbsp. peanut butter, 1/2 banana, 1 cup almond milk @ 7:00 a.m.— in a rush to get to work
Breakfast	
Snack	

Lunch	
Snack	
Dinner	
Snack	

A Day of Healthy Eating

This is what a day of healthy eating might look like. This meal plan provides about 1500 calories distributed in this manner: 95 grams of protein for muscle building and tissue repair, 170 grams of energy-giving carbohydrates, 50 grams of healthy fats and 30–35 grams of dietary fibre.

Breakfast	1/2 cup oats, 1/2 tsp. cinnamon, 1 cup strawberries, 1 tbsp. ground flax seeds, 1 cup almond milk, 1 boiled egg
Snack	1 apple, 12 almonds
Lunch	3 oz. chicken breast, 2 cups salad (mixed greens, tomato, cucumber), 1/4 cup chickpeas, 1 tbsp. homemade vinaigrette
Snack	2 celery stalks, 6 baby carrots, 2 tbsp. guacamole, 2 slices of light rye crispbread
Dinner	4 oz. white fish (cod or sole) cooked with 1 tsp. coconut oil, 1/2 cup brown rice, 1 cup broccoli
Snack	3/4 cup (6 oz.) Greek yogurt (non-fat, plain), 1 tbsp. almond butter or tahini (sesame seed butter)

For vegetarians or for those following a vegan diet, there are many sources of plant-based protein. Meat and dairy can be replaced with a variety of beans and lentils, nuts and seeds and their butters, quinoa, eda-mame beans, tofu, tempeh, vegetarian meat products, soy milk, almond or coconut yogurt, and vegan protein powders and bars.

Recipes

Here are a few vegetable dip and salad dressing recipes that will make increasing your vegetable intake very enjoyable.

Homemade Vinaigrette

Ingredients:

- 1/3 cup extra-virgin olive oil
- 1/3 cup balsamic vinegar or red wine vinegar
- pinch of sea salt
- freshly ground pepper to taste

Place ingredients in a glass jar with a tight-fitting lid and shake. This mixture is safe to store on the counter for a few days. Once you add fresh ingredients such as garlic, fresh herbs, mustard or yogurt, it will need to be refrigerated. Leave to stand at room temperature for 30 minutes before use, as it may solidify once refrigerated. By making it fresh every time, you can avoid this inconvenience.

To create a different flavour, add:

1 tsp. Italian seasoning
1 tsp. minced garlic

For a creamier dressing, add:

2 tbsp. plain yogurt or 1 tsp. prepared mustard

Basic Guacamole

Ingredients:

- 2 ripe avocados
- pinch of sea salt

Cut the avocados in half; remove the skin and seed. Place the avocados in a bowl with a pinch of sea salt. Mash lightly with a fork.

For extra flavour, add:

1 clove of minced garlic
1 chopped tomato
1 chopped green onion
juice from 1 lime
freshly ground pepper to taste

Simple Hummus or White Bean Dip

Ingredients:

- 1 can chickpeas (400 mL, or 14 ounces; reserve some of the liquid to add to the mixture to achieve desired consistency)
- juice from 1 lemon
- 1 clove of minced garlic
- 2 tbsp. tahini
- 1 tbsp. olive oil
- 1 tsp. sea salt
- freshly ground pepper to taste

For white bean dip, replace chickpeas with cannellini beans and leave out the tahini.

Blend until creamy in a high-powered blender or food processor. Place in a glass container and store in the refrigerator.

Bone Health

Bone health is of great concern for most women as they near menopause. As you age, you may be more at risk of developing osteoporosis, a thinning of the bones that can increase your risk of fractures.

After you reach menopause, your doctor will send you for a bone density test. This is a non-invasive procedure that uses a low-dose X-ray over your hips and spine to measure the amount of mineral in your bones. This tool helps you and your doctor find out where you stand in regards to bone health. It also provides a baseline to which subsequent tests will be compared.

If bone health is a concern for you, it is never too late to improve your condition.

Ways to Improve Bone Health

Lifestyle and nutrition are very important to bone health. Smoking, drinking, being too skinny, lacking physical activity and eating poorly contribute to bone loss. By age 30, bone mass has reached its peak. If you are in your 40s and 50s, here are some nutrition-based suggestions to help prevent bone loss and increase your chances of maintaining bone health as you age.

Calcium

The National Osteoporosis Foundation recommends 1000 mg of calcium daily from food and supplements for women 50 and younger and 1200 mg for women over 51. Food labels are based on Daily Value (DV) of 1000 mg, therefore, be aware that if the label says that this food provides 30 % DV of calcium, this is equivalent to 300 mg of calcium. Check with your doctor to see if you require supplementation.

Calcium-rich Foods

We traditionally think of dairy as our go-to source for calcium. In a world where many people have food intolerances or are averse to dairy, it is good to have other options for calcium-rich foods.

Note: Pasteurization of milk and milk products diminishes the available calcium.

Here is a list of non-dairy foods rich in absorbable calcium.

- **Beans:** edamame beans, tofu, white beans and navy beans
- **Enriched beverages:** almond milk, rice milk and other calcium-enriched non-dairy milk beverages
- **Fish:** canned salmon and sardines with bones
- **Fruit:** oranges, dried figs and dried apricots
- **Grains:** oats and quinoa
- **Leafy greens:** broccoli, kale, collard greens and dark green lettuce; spinach and swiss chard are great leafy greens, but they are high in oxalates, which render the calcium less available
- **Nuts and seeds:** almonds and almond butter, brazil nuts, chia seeds, sesame seeds and tahini, and sunflower seeds

Vitamin D

Most people in Canada and the United States do not get enough of this "sunshine" vitamin. Osteoporosis Canada states that vitamin D is essential for the treatment of osteoporosis because it promotes calcium absorption from the diet and is necessary for normal bone growth. The new guidelines recommend daily supplementation of 400–1000 IU for adults under age 50 without osteoporosis or conditions affecting vitamin D absorption. For adults over 50, supplements of between 800–2000 IU are recommended. Doses above that require medical supervision. Check with your doctor to see how much vitamin D you should be taking.

Eliminate Addictive Substances, Soft Drinks and Salt (Sodium)

Reduce or eliminate caffeine, alcohol, nicotine, soft drinks and salt from your diet. These have a negative effect on bone health by either promoting calcium excretion from your bones or preventing calcium absorption.

Maintain Acid/Alkaline Balance

For survival, your body will always try to maintain its acid/alkaline (pH) balance. Our Western diet is rich in processed foods, sugar, dairy and meat—all of which are acidic. In this environment, your body tries to return to a healthy pH level by leaching calcium from the bones in order to buffer this extra acidity.

To maintain a healthy acid/alkaline balance, include more alkaline foods in your diet. Leafy green vegetables, sprouts and berries are some of the most alkaline foods.

Heart Health

Heart disease used to be regarded as a man's disease. But the Heart and Stroke Foundation quotes that Statistics Canada for 2008 show that 29.7 percent of all female deaths were due to heart disease.

More and more women, especially after menopause, are at risk for heart disease. Estrogen has a positive effect on the flexibility of your arteries as well as helping maintain healthy cholesterol levels. Therefore, the drop in estrogen after menopause may be one of the risk factors for heart disease. Other risk factors include being overweight, eating a high-fat diet, smoking, being inactive, having high cholesterol, high blood pressure, diabetes or a family history of heart disease. Visit your doctor to have a heart health check-up. Have them check your blood pressure and cholesterol levels. Discuss what your personal risk factors may be.

Here is a 2015 update on the statistics for heart disease and stroke by the American Heart Association.

- Heart disease is the number one killer of women, and it is more deadly than all forms of cancer combined.
- While 1 in 31 American women dies from breast cancer each year, 1 in 3 dies of heart disease.
- Heart disease causes 1 in 3 women's deaths each year, killing approximately one woman every minute.
- Only 1 in 5 American women believe that heart disease is her greatest health threat.
- An estimated 43 million women in the United States are affected by heart disease.
- Ninety percent of women have one or more risk factors for developing heart disease.
- Since 1984, more women than men have died each year from heart disease.

Heart-healthy Food

Nutrition plays an important role in minimizing the risk factors for heart disease. Here are some heart-healthy foods you should be including in your daily diet.

- **Beans and lentils:** Include more beans and lentils in your diet. These are high in heart-healthy fibre and protein, and they are low in fat.

- **Fish:** Fatty fish such as salmon, trout, fresh tuna, mackerel and sardines are high in omega-3 fatty acids that are beneficial for the heart. Eat two servings a week.

- **Fresh fruits and vegetables:** Enjoy six or more servings a day. These foods contain little or no fat, are low in calories, are high in heart-healthy fibre, and are rich in vitamins and minerals that help to protect against heart disease.

- **Grains:** Whole grains such as brown rice, buckwheat, millet, oats, quinoa, rye and wheat are rich in heart-healthy fibre and have a host of other important nutrients necessary for overall health. Eat two to three servings a day.

- **Herbs and spices:** Use flavourful herbs and spices instead of salt to season your food.

- **Lean meat:** Skinless chicken and turkey, white fish and shellfish are great sources of lean protein. Eat one or two small (3 oz.) servings a day.

- **Nuts and seeds:** A small handful of nuts or seeds, or two tablespoons of nut or seed butter, is a great high-fibre snack and a source of healthy fats.

- **Oils and fats:** Here are some good oils and fats that help protect the heart and support overall health. Remember that all fats, whether healthy or not, are high in calories. Eat in moderation.

  Good for cooking at high heat: virgin coconut oil, avocado oil, almond oil

  Good for light to medium heat (sautéing): olive oil, pastured butter, sesame seed oil, walnut oil

  Good for salad dressings, dips, added to cooked dishes, or taken straight from a tablespoon: flax seed oil, hemp seed oil, hazelnut oil, olive oil

Foods to Avoid

When it comes to heart health, there are some foods that can be detrimental to your health. Limit the following foods.

- **High-fat meat and animal products:** Bacon, sausages, beef and full-fat dairy products

- **Salt (sodium):** Can be found in deli meats, condiments, salad dressings, processed foods and snack foods.

- **Sugar:** Table sugar and products that contain added sugar: processed foods, snack foods, store-bought juices, salad dressings, sauces, soft drinks, candy, jams, boxed cereal and canned fruit.

- **Trans fats, hydrogenated/partially hydrogenated fats:** These fats elevate your bad cholesterol (LDL) and can lower your good cholesterol (HDL). Avoid margarine, shortening, fried foods, processed foods and baked goods from the store.

Mental Health

Depression affects many women in mid-life; it is twice more prevalent in women than in men. The change in hormone levels as you near menopause is one of the most common factors that may precipitate depression. These physical changes often have an emotional consequence. Depression can manifest as:

- Anxiety
- Hopelessness
- Insomnia
- Loss of interest in activities one used to enjoy
- Sadness
- Self-hatred
- Tiredness
- Unfounded guilt
- Weight gain due to eating in an attempt to feel better
- Weight loss due to lack of appetite

Stress management and physical exercise have enormous beneficial effects on improving mental well-being. Proper nutrition plays a very important role as well.

> " Making a change with my diet
> changed my whole life. "
> —Donna J. Dingwall

Donna J. Dingwall, age 55, has struggled with depression for a long time. Her troubles began when she was a little girl. It wasn't until she hit the age of 40 that things started to improve because she made some important dietary changes. If you struggle with depression, my hope is that you can draw some inspiration from Donna's account.

I grew up with an abusive, alcoholic father. By the time I was 14, I weighed 210 pounds. I had always been an emotional eater because of the abuse. At this point I decided to starve myself for a whole year, eating only 150 calories a day. My diet consisted of cup-a-soup and Melba toast. I had an eating disorder!

I managed to lose 90 pounds. I had just started my period, and then I lost my weight so fast that it stopped. I was concerned, so I went to see my doctor. He noticed that I had lost a lot of weight and was really happy for me. He said, "Whatever you're doing, keep it up!" He didn't even ask what I was doing. Unfortunately, losing all that weight drew more attention to me. I got abused even more, so over time I gained the weight back.

I had been in several abusive situations, and as a young mom in my 30s, I had to seek refuge in a homeless shelter just to feel safe. I fell into deep depression. I had a 2-year-old son and a 2-week-old baby boy.

I felt I was back on my feet. Unfortunately, two years later I found myself in a homeless shelter for a second time in my life, and I wound up even more depressed.

I was in the shelter for two weeks, and in that whole time, I managed to sleep for seven hours in total. I was a wreck! It was then that I went to my doctor about my depression. I got sleeping pills, antidepressants, thyroid medication and medication for my attention deficit disorder. I was on all of this for quite a while.

A friend I had known since I was 19 could see that I was really depressed, and she suggested I read a book by Dr. Kathleen DesMaisons, *The Sugar Addict's Total Recovery Program*. I was 40 years old by now. I resisted at first. When I finally read it, it was like I was reading my own story. It was amazing! At this point I was so pitifully sad that I even went as far as thinking that I would gladly give up my right arm if I could experience some happiness in my life. The only thing that kept me going was my children. I did not have any other reason to live.

Dr. Kathleen DesMaisons's book is all about nutrition and changing your lifestyle. I realized that I had been eating wrong ever since my childhood. The book goes through a seven-step program. I followed the seven steps, and it took me a year to get through all of them. I was so determined to not feel so sad anymore that changing my lifestyle did not seem hard at all. I had my little boys, and I had to be a mom for them. I didn't want to live in this depressed state anymore.

Making a change with my diet changed my whole life. The first thing Kathleen teaches in her book is eating breakfast within one hour of waking up—a breakfast that contains an adequate amount of protein. The next thing is slowly changing your whites to browns. For example, having brown rice instead of the traditional white. Next is giving up sugar. Let me emphasize that this is not a weight-loss program; it's a way to get you off these addictive substances. Most people who are not health conscious are addicted to sugar or whites. When I heightened my awareness of sugars in food and started reading labels, sugar was in everything, and I had to give up so much. I was fine with it though. I was ready!

My body started to change. I started to lose weight. When I began following the seven-step program in the book, I was 200 pounds. I now weigh 132 pounds! Another success was slowly going off all medication. I worked closely with my doctor to achieve this. I felt like a million bucks! For the first time in my children's lives, they saw their mom smile and laugh!

Donna and I spoke at length about her journey out of depression. Nutrition definitely played an important part, but there was more. As we sat in her in-home workout room, I looked around at all the equipment she had gathered over the years and asked, "Would you say that exercise has been beneficial to your mental state?"

Absolutely! Right now, exercise is my drug of choice. Look around at this workout room. This is my therapy room. I can jump on the rebounder for a little bit. Run on my treadmill. Do some yoga. Lift some weights. In order to maintain my healthy mental state and to physically feel better, I have to exercise. But you know what? I want to exercise because it makes me feel so good!

It's exciting for me to feel good, and I want to share that with other women. I am now a health coach, encouraging women over 40 to get and stay fit. I also help them with their mental state, because I have been there. I have been obese, and I have had an eating disorder. I have been abused, and I have been depressed. I have been through a lot of things in my life, and I can relate to pretty much anything that anyone could share. I want to encourage women who are at 200 pounds that it is possible. I am living proof. It's a lifestyle change. You can't go back to the way you were, because then you go back to being bigger, depressed or whatever state you were in. I refuse to go back there!

Help Yourself with Food

As illustrated in Donna's story, food can affect your mental health and your mood. You cannot deprive your body of macronutrients (protein, carbohydrates, and fats) and micronutrients (vitamins and minerals) and yet expect it to function optimally. Eating a nutrient-dense diet is the foundation of well-being, both physical and mental.

Here are some foods to include in your daily diet.

- **B-complex vitamins:** The vitamins in the B group support and maintain the health of your nervous system, in particular vitamins B-12 and B-9 (otherwise known as folate in foods, or folic acid in vitamin form). Research continues to find a correlation between the deficiency in B vitamins and depression. Vitamins B-12 and B-9 show promise in helping to manage depression.

  Food sources of B-12 include animal products such as dairy, fish, poultry, eggs and beef. Vegetarian sources of this vitamin can be found in non-dairy milks and breakfast cereals fortified with B-12.

  B-9 (folate) can be found in foods such as a variety of beans and lentils, as well as in vegetables such as asparagus, broccoli, Brussels sprouts, cauliflower and dark leafy greens.

  Talk to your doctor to see if you should be taking a B-complex vitamin supplement.

- **Complex carbohydrates:** They help to stabilize your blood sugar levels and prompt the release of serotonin, a brain chemical that has a positive effect on mood. Serotonin is sometimes called the "happiness" hormone. Include more whole grain foods in your diet such as oats, brown rice, quinoa, whole grain bread and pasta, as well as sweet potato, squash, beans and lentils, and vegetables and fruits.

- **Omega-3 fatty acids:** This type of fat supports brain function and has a positive effect on mood. Scientists agree that consuming foods rich in omega-3 fatty acids can elevate mood, prevent depression and reduce the symptoms of depression. Some omega-3 foods include fatty fish such as salmon and sardines, flax seed oil, and nuts and seeds such as almonds, pecans, walnuts, ground flax seeds, chia seeds and pumpkin seeds.

- **Tryptophan:** Eating foods high in tryptophan is a natural way to help boost serotonin production. Your body utilizes tryptophan in order to make serotonin. Animal protein sources such as turkey, fish, beef, chicken and eggs are high in tryptophan, as are foods from the plant kingdom such as chia seeds, sesame seeds, ground flax seeds, almonds and spirulina. Eat tryptophan foods in combination with complex carbohydrates for best results. In addition, tryptophan foods also contain amino acids, the building blocks of protein; these help with mental acuity and alertness.

- **Vitamin D:** This vitamin, called the "sunshine" vitamin, is often thought of in relation to bone health, but it is also showing promise in studies related to depression. Vitamin D is produced when the skin is exposed to sunlight. Unfortunately, many of us live in a climate where we are covered up for months of the year—and then when it warms up, we cover our skin with sunscreen. Our skin is seldom exposed to sunlight. For this reason, many of us are deficient in vitamin D. Although this vitamin is best obtained by being outdoors, it is also found in milk and non-dairy milk beverages that are fortified with vitamin D. Talk to your doctor to see if you should take a vitamin D supplement.

Digestive Health

Good digestion helps support a healthy colon and is essential in helping you absorb the various beneficial nutrients from your diet. As you age, your stomach acid, which is responsible for digestion, is diminished. The production of hydrochloric acid (HCL), your natural stomach acid, begins to decrease. Age, stress, eating too much in one sitting and eating too much junk food are some of the common factors that contribute to poor digestion.

Symptoms of Poor Digestion

Some of the most common symptoms of poor digestion are:

- Bad breath
- Bloating after meals
- Body odour
- Burping after meals
- Chronic constipation
- Feeling tired after a meal
- Finding undigested food in your stool
- Heartburn
- Heavy feeling after a meal
- Passing gas after meals

Ways to Improve Digestion

We have talked about foods and supplements to help improve your hormone balance, manage your weight and enhance your bone, heart and mental health. But without proper digestion, these wonderful nutrients will not be digested, absorbed and utilized by your body. Most of the beneficial nutrients you ingest will be going to waste.

Here are some changes you can implement to help you improve your digestion, allowing you to utilize your food more efficiently.

- **Eat until you are satisfied, but not full:** You know what full feels like, because you would have experienced that feeling at Thanksgiving, Christmas or at an all-you-can-eat buffet. That should never be your goal. Leave the table when you still have enough room to eat more (75 percent full). This leaves enough room for the digestive process to take place. Eat smaller meals more often throughout the day.

- **Eat slowly:** They say that it takes 20 minutes for your brain to register that your stomach is full. Eating slowly will accomplish two things: One, you will not overeat, and two, eating in a mindful fashion will improve digestion. Eating while rushed or stressed will shut down the digestive process. Eat in a relaxed state and truly take time to appreciate your food.

- **Take time to chew your food properly:** If you are following the "eat slowly" suggestion, you are probably already adopting this principle. Chewing your food thoroughly will help break it down into smaller particles; this lightens the load on the digestive process. Also, the more chewing you do, the more saliva is produced to help break down the food.

- **Don't drink too much water during meals:** You should drink lots of water throughout the day. Keeping hydrated all day long will improve your overall digestion when it comes to mealtime. But if you are having trouble with digestion, it is recommended that you only have small sips of room-temperature water during your meal so that stomach acids will not become diluted. Drink your water 30 minutes before a meal. Don't drink ice-cold water because this will diminish digestion. The only time you should drink cold water is while exercising or during a hot flash episode, in order to cool yourself.

- **Limit dietary fat:** Deep-fried foods, red meat and full-fat dairy can be difficult to digest and can slow down your digestion. Eliminate deep-fried foods from your diet. Red meat can be

replaced with chicken, turkey, lean cuts of pork or f
general is difficult to digest. If you still wish to enjo
choose low-fat options.

- **Reduce processed foods:** They are generally laden w
salt, fat and chemicals. These are hard on the digestive sy
can cause heartburn, gas, bloating and dehydration as yo
attempts to process them. Choose fresh, whole foods in

- **Eat high-fibre foods:** Foods high in fibre help keep your
moving properly so that digestion and elimination func
their best. Fruits and vegetables should be eaten daily.
high-fibre foods are whole grains, nuts and seeds, and bean
lentils.

- **Include probiotics:** This good bacteria helps keep the dige
system healthy. Look for food with live and active cultures
as yogurt and kefir. Other foods with probiotics are miso and
erkraut. Probiotics also come in supplement form. Talk to yo
doctor to see if a probiotic supplement is right for you.

- **Take digestive enzymes:** Sometimes the digestive system nee
a little boost with extra digestive enzymes in supplement form
These will help break down and assimilate nutrients from th
food you eat.

- **Be physically active:** Being physically active is essential to general health and well-being. It is also beneficial to your digestive
health. It increases peristaltic movement, which keeps food moving through your system, preventing constipation and bloating.

See chapter 4 on the importance of exercise. It includes an illustrated
workout routine.

Try one or more of these suggestions to help you improve your digestion.
If you have not been able to improve your digestion and eliminate certain

uncomfortable symptoms with these suggestions, talk to a healthcare professional who can test you for food allergies. A food allergy can derail even your best efforts to improve digestive health.

Measure Your Digestive Transit Time

Once you have taken steps to improve your digestion, you can do a simple at-home test to see how effective your digestive system is. Transit time refers to how long it takes for your food to travel from your mouth, move through your digestive tract, and be eliminated from your body. In a person with a healthy digestive system, it should take 12–24 hours for this process. Anything beyond 24 hours shows that you are not processing your food at a healthy rate. Food is staying in your colon too long; this causes putrefaction and a build-up of toxins that can lead to disease.

The test consists of eating a cup of corn or fresh beets, or 2 tablespoons of sesame seeds. Watch to see how long it takes for the corn, red dye from the beets or for the sesame seeds to appear in your stool. If it takes longer than 24 hours, please review the section earlier in this chapter called "What Is Fibre?" You may be struggling with constipation and should add more fibre to your diet.

Food Preparation Made Easy

> " Nutrition is the key ingredient to a
> successful healthy lifestyle. "
> —Carla Hampshire

People tell me that they wish they could eat healthier, but they don't have the time. Here are some practical ideas to help make food preparation easier.

Having the right equipment makes food preparation less time consuming. Here are some basic items you should have in your kitchen.

- Appropriate sized pots and pans
- Blender
- Cookie sheet
- Cutting board
- Electric grill
- Food processor
- Food scale
- Glass salad and mixing bowls
- Glass storage containers
- Hand mixer
- Juicer
- Kitchen knives
- Measuring cups and spoons
- Rice cooker
- Two 9" by 13" pans
- Vegetable steamer

How to Grocery Shop

Buy it fresh, and prepare it yourself!

Plan your meals ahead of time, and prepare a standard shopping list. Use Saturday as a food preparation day. Here is a sample shopping list.

Healthy Eating Grocery List

Fruit	Vegetables	Whole Grains
Apples	Asparagus	Barley
Bananas	Beets	Brown rice
Berries	Broccoli	Buckwheat
Kiwi	Carrots	Oats
Lemons	Cauliflower	Quinoa
Melons	Celery	Whole grain bread
Oranges	Cucumber	Whole grain crackers

Pears	Green beans	Whole grain pasta
	Leafy greens	
	Zucchini	

Meat and Other Protein	Starchy Vegetables	Dairy and Alternatives
Chicken	Beans and lentils	Almond milk
Eggs	Corn	Cottage cheese
Protein powder	Peas	Goat cheese
Salmon	Potatoes	Greek yogurt
Shellfish	Pumpkin	
Tofu	Squash	
Turkey	Turnips	
White fish	Yams	

Healthy Fats		Condiments
Avocados		Apple cider vinegar
Coconut oil		Balsamic vinegar
Nuts, seeds and their		Herbs and spices
butters		Honey
Olive oil		Mustard
		Salsa

Additional Shopping Tips

- In the produce aisle, shop for fruits and vegetables that are fresh and firm, preferably produce that is in season. Choose organic produce as much as possible; it is not always more expensive. Look for farmers' markets in your neighbourhood. Remember that fresh is always more nutritious than frozen, but frozen is always a better choice than canned.

- In the meat department, shop for lean cuts of fresh meat and fish. With poultry, buy skinless cuts or remove the skin before cooking.

- Limit the consumption of foods that come in a box, bag or can. Processed foods lack nutrient value.

- Shop for a variety of spices. Healthy food does not have to be tasteless and boring. Spice up your food with basil, black pepper, cayenne pepper, cumin, dill, garlic, ginger, marjoram, mint, onion, oregano, parsley, rosemary, sage, sea salt, thyme, turmeric and more.

Meal Preparation Ideas

- Boil 6–12 eggs and keep them in the refrigerator. Boiled eggs make a great protein snack.

- Wash and cut your vegetables, and store them in the refrigerator. Your vegetables will then be ready to be used in salads, soups, stews and stir-fry recipes. They also make a great grab-and-go snack.

- Make a large pot of vegetable soup, stew or stir-fry. Store one portion in the refrigerator and the rest in the freezer. You can easily add some cubed chicken breast to this now, or add it in later when you are ready to serve the meal.

- Cook multiple chicken breasts (oven-roasted, grilled or barbequed) and refrigerate them. These are great as part of a meal, as a healthy protein snack or added to soups, stews and other recipes.

- Cook a large Sunday meal so that you have leftovers for Monday lunch or dinner.

- Use your rice cooker to prepare a large amount of brown rice or quinoa. Store in the refrigerator. It is great as a side dish, or to add variety and nutrition to a salad, soup, stew or stir-fry.

> " Take care of your body. It's the
> only place you have to live. "
> —Jim Rohn

CHAPTER 4

The Importance of Exercise

" When you exercise your body feels so good.
It's happy. It's like a well-tuned guitar. "
—Christina Ryan

We often associate exercise with weight loss, but exercise goes well beyond that. There is no lack of evidence to show that regular physical activity is essential to the well-being of the human body. It is one of the most important things you can do to maintain good physical and mental health as you age. Research suggests that staying active may reduce your risk of having heart disease, a stroke, some cancers, type 2 diabetes and other conditions.

As you get older, your metabolism slows down, your hormone levels may become unbalanced and your bone density and your muscle mass decrease. Your weight and blood pressure increase. You become more prone to obesity, heart disease, mental health issues and osteoporosis. Exercise is one of your best friends when it comes to mitigating these issues.

Exercise Helps with Weight Management

If you are overweight, you know it by how you look and feel, by how your clothes fit, by that dreaded number on the scale or because your doctor told you so. No matter how you look at it, if you need to lose weight, exercise should be an important part of your overall wellness plan. Here is an accurate way of determining whether you are overweight.

Calculating Your Body Mass Index

The body mass index (BMI) is a number calculated from your weight and height. It is one way to determine if you are at a healthy weight. The Centers for Disease Control and Prevention state that BMI can be used to screen for weight categories that may lead to health problems. You can manually calculate your BMI in the following manner, or look to the chart below.

Imperial Formula:
BMI = (Weight in Pounds / (Height in inches × Height in inches)) × 703

Metric Formula:
BMI = Weight in kilograms / (Height in metres × Height in metres)

For example, if you weigh 165 pounds and are 5'2" (62") tall, you would calculate your BMI in the following manner: (165/ (62 × 62)) × 703 = 30.2

According to this chart, with a BMI of over 30, you would be classified as obese.

BMI	Classification
< 18.5	Underweight
18.5–24.9	Ideal BMI
25–29.9	Overweight
> 30	Obese
> 35	Severely obese
> 40	Morbidly obese

In the following chart, you can find your BMI without having to do the math. Look for your height in feet in the left-hand column, and then find your weight in pounds from the top row. Your BMI is where the two points meet. Compare your result with the BMI classification above.

Finding Your BMI

Weight (lbs)

Height (feet)	120	130	140	150	160	170	180	190	200	210	220
5'0"	23	25	27	29	31	32	35	37	39	41	43
5'1"	23	25	26	28	30	32	34	36	38	40	42
5'2"	22	24	25	27	29	31	33	35	37	38	40
5'3"	21	23	25	27	28	30	32	34	36	37	39
5'4"	21	22	24	26	28	29	31	33	34	36	38
5'5"	20	22	23	25	27	28	30	32	33	35	37
5'6"	19	21	23	24	26	27	29	31	32	34	36
5'7"	19	20	22	24	25	27	28	30	31	33	35
5'8"	18	20	21	23	24	26	27	29	30	32	34
5'9"	18	19	21	22	24	25	27	28	30	31	33
5'10"	17	19	20	22	23	24	26	27	29	30	32

For an automatic calculation of your BMI, you can also go to www. bmi-calculator.net.

Take a moment now to find your body mass index. How did you rate? If your BMI is above 25, keep gathering the helpful tools this book offers. Commit to making lifestyle changes that will improve your health and well-being.

Data from the National Health and Nutrition Examination Survey (2009–2010) states that:

- More than 2 in 3 adults are considered to be overweight or obese.
- More than 1 in 3 adults are considered to be obese.
- More than 1 in 20 adults are considered to have extreme obesity.

These statistics are very alarming. One of the reasons for this rise in obesity is the lack of physical activity. We have become a sedentary people.

If we look back one or two generations, obesity was not prevalent. Our grandmothers and great-grandmothers worked hard all day long; their level of daily physical activity was quite elevated. They worked on the farm, did laundry by hand, fetched water, cut firewood, cooked from scratch and even sewed their own clothes. This was their exercise.

We live in an automated world where physical activity has been significantly diminished. We drive everywhere, and we sit at our jobs for hours on end. When we come home, we sit again in front of the television or computer. Because of this lack of activity, over time our bodies become weak. Our heart and lungs are not challenged. Our muscles lose their tone. As the old adage goes, "Use it or lose it!" Our bodies are meant to be active. We have to find ways to include physical activity into our daily lives.

I spoke with Charmaine Ironside, personal trainer and owner of Ironside Fitness. She has worked with many clients over the years, helping them get in the best shape of their lives. This is what her clients report to her.

> My clients over 40 often say that something does shift around this time. Many women notice that they have more of an uphill battle in terms of maintaining a healthy weight. By adding fitness into their life three days a week or more, it makes such a big difference. For many of our clients, it has become a way of life.

> When they first came to me, they couldn't imagine doing this long-term; they simply wanted to reach a weight-loss goal. Now, three years later, the same clients say that they will never leave.

As you read the following story, I hope it gives you the motivation you need to get started with your own exercise plan.

Nearing 40, Christina Ryan realized that she was on a downward spiral. She was overweight, was eating all the wrong foods and hadn't exercised in far too long. She finally found the motivation to regain control of her health. This is her inspiring story.

My lifestyle is very busy. I am a 40-year-old mom of two. I work in the media as a photojournalist and videographer, and my working schedule is always different. You never know what assignments you're working on, or where you're going. On top of that, my younger daughter was born with Down's syndrome and has a very complicated medical history. She is 16 years old now, so I have been putting myself on the back burner for quite some time. I was smoking and not eating very healthy, and I certainly wasn't exercising. I weighed 190 pounds and was wearing a size 14.

When I was 39, I finally realized that I was either going to have to jump off a bridge, or I'd have to start taking better care of myself. With my daughter being disabled, I know that I will be caring for her for a long time. I realized that I wasn't in any shape to look after anybody, and I needed to make changes in my life. When you don't exercise and don't do anything for yourself, you get lazier, and it's harder to begin activities. I didn't want to be that way anymore. I wanted to be healthy and happy.

The key thing for me was starting to exercise. When I first started out, I did not want to go to a gym because I knew that I would not be able to keep up. With my daughter's disability, she needs care at home, and I can't always find people to come in and look after her. I needed an exercise regimen that I could keep up with, and that I could do at home. I started doing walking programs. They made me feel good! I found that I was craving exercise, and I could see the weight coming off. I was getting slimmer—it was so exciting!

Then my friend took me out to go mountain climbing. So I climbed a mountain, and I nearly died! But the smell of the pines and being out in the forest—it was so fabulous! I started climbing a mountain once or twice a week all by myself. Then I started challenging myself to see how fast I could go up. The demands it made on my body were incredible; I could feel it in my legs. It was sweet agony. The more changes I saw in my body, the more excited I got. I pushed myself more and started doing activities I never thought I would do.

I rock climb now, and I joined a basketball team. I went from someone who used to sit on the couch, watch TV and eat really nasty things to treating my body more like a person—more like how I wanted to be treated. I am now down to 153 pounds and am wearing a size 8, and I'm still going strong. I quit smoking and stopped drinking coffee, and I traded in my candy for healthier food choices.

Before, it was so hard to get out of bed. Now there's a bounce in my step, and I feel younger! When you exercise, your body feels so good. It's happy! It's like a well-tuned guitar.

Christina is a busy woman. By committing to exercise, she was able to lose weight. But even more important, she regained her health, vitality and energy.

I challenge you to include more physical activity into your day. Later on in this chapter, you will be invited to try out a simple workout program that you can do at home. It requires no equipment, just a little bit of commitment on your part.

Exercise Slows Down the Aging Process

> " Those who think they have no time
> for bodily exercise will sooner or later
> have to find time for illness. "
> —Edward Stanley

Disuse versus Aging

Are you beginning to feel old? Are you experiencing a decline in your physical performance? Although aging is a natural biological process, the decrease in functional ability is mostly associated with disuse. When you fail to do something that you are able to do and that you ought to do, you will eventually have less capacity to do it. You may not have the power to stop Father Time or control Mother Nature, but you can use exercise to slow down aging—and in some cases, you can reverse it.

It is common to accept physical decline as a normal part of aging. The fact is that if you are not involved in some form of physical activity on a daily basis, you will gradually lose your natural abilities and your health, and you will soon begin to look and feel old.

The Benefits of Exercise as a Woman Ages

Exercise is one of the most effective ways to slow down the aging process, and it can improve your quality of life at any age. Including physical activity in your daily routine can help you maintain your independence as you age and increase your ability to live a life free of chronic disease, pain and disability. The range of health benefits attributed to physical activity are numerous. A well-rounded exercise regime will include strength training, cardiovascular exercise, balance exercises and flexibility training.

Strength training will improve both strength and function of the muscles, helping you perform daily activities with greater ease. Bone density and joint function are also improved, reducing the risk of debilitating conditions such as osteoporosis and arthritis. With strength training, flexibility and balance are also enhanced; this can lessen the probability of falls and the resulting disability.

Cardiovascular exercise, though often associated with weight loss, also has the benefit of keeping your heart, lungs and bones healthy and strong, and it helps the thyroid gland to function optimally. Walking, running, hiking, dancing, tennis and other weight-bearing forms of exercise are excellent examples of cardiovascular exercise. Swimming, though a great form of cardiovascular exercise, does not benefit the bones in the same way because it is not a weight-bearing exercise.

> **Exercise may be the closest thing
> to the fountain of youth.**
> —Carla Hampshire

Imagine joining a gym at the age of 80. This is exactly what Roberta Jorgensen decided to do. What was Roberta's motivation? To fit into a dress for her daughter's wedding. Now at age 87, she reports all kinds of benefits she has gained by including physical activity in her life. "I feel less tired, I can walk faster and I can put on my socks without struggling. I can shovel my walk, and I even carry a 20-pound bag of kitty litter from my car to my basement without too much effort." Yes, 87-year-old Roberta still drives!

Let's review the benefits Roberta experienced by starting to exercise. Not only did she trim her waistline, but she felt energized, improved her cardiovascular endurance, became more flexible and increased her strength.

She often laughs at the fact that she waited until she was 80 to take up exercise. With her new-found energy, she fulfilled a lifelong dream of taking a cruise to Tahiti. Roberta is living proof that it is never too late to get started.

Exercise can improve:

- Balance, flexibility and posture
- Bone density and joint function

- Cardiovascular endurance, muscular strength and weight management
- Cognitive function, psychological health and sleep

> " If we could give every individual the right amount of nourishment and exercise, not too little and not too much, we would have found the safest way to health. "
> —Hippocrates

John Stanton is the founder of the Running Room, with 130 locations in Canada and the United States. He is also the author of 10 books on running and walking. I knew he would have some excellent insight on the topic of exercise. This is what he shared with me during our interview.

You can go on any healthcare website—it doesn't matter which one. It could be heart and stroke, breast cancer, arthritis or diabetes. They are all recommending the same thing, and that is—choose your nutrition well. By eating more wholesome foods, especially fruits and vegetables, and combining that with the routine of exercise, I think we can push back the clock.

The best place to begin is with one of the most simplistic exercises; it's also the number one exercise in North America, and it's the most underrated exercise of all: walking. Often when a person first starts to think of exercising—and I was one of them—it's the fear that keeps you from starting. If you put on your sneakers and your jogging suit and start jogging through your neighbourhood, you're going to be very self-conscious and embarrassed when you are out there. Whereas if you go out and walk, nobody pays attention to you at all. That's a good place to begin.

If you can spend four or five weeks doing what I call preconditioning, which is just walking, and work your way up to 45 minutes of walking, it's an amazing precursor. Then you can take up running, if that's your choice. But preconditioning is so important.

When I started the Running Room in the early 1980s, running was a male-dominated sport. Today, if you go to any of the major races, you will see that it is dominated by women. Women have taken a leading position in the running community. I think they have done it for a number of reasons. One, it fits their busy schedules. Two, it's social. Women have brought more of a social component to running than there was before.

When people start a running program, I always say to keep three things in mind.

- Keep it gentle enough so that you don't get injured and stay highly motivated.
- Keep it progressive; in other words you do not want it so gentle that you don't see any improvements.
- Keep it fun, otherwise you won't do it.

You have to find something that appeals to you. Running and walking appeals to a lot of people because it caters to their busy schedules. People are busy today no matter who you are. The best thing about a running or walking program is that you can go out and run or walk at any time of day. You can go in the early morning or late at night. You can do it alone, or you can do it in a group. I highly recommend getting in a group because the buddy system keeps you honest. There is that positive peer pressure that comes from it.

At the Running Room, the way we start people is we have them run for a minute, walk for a minute. We have them doing that six times the first week, and they do it every other day. Then in week two, we encourage them to run for two minutes and walk for one minute. Do another six sets of that. Then in week three, do three minutes of running and one minute of walking. By the end of 10 weeks, they are doing 10 minutes of running and one minute of walking. They can then continue with their running and jogging program, or they can go on and run a 5K or 10K race if they decide that running is going to be their option.

So keep it gentle, keep it progressive and keep it fun!

How to Stay Physically Active as You Age

We are all at different levels of fitness. Respect your current level of fitness, and determine to improve upon it. If you have not exercised for some time, or if you have health concerns such as heart trouble, high blood pressure, diabetes or obesity, talk to your doctor before starting a new exercise routine.

Daily physical activity will help improve your heart health, strengthen your bones, keep your lungs strong, improve your sleep, manage your weight and stress, and help reduce your risk of disease.

The National Center for Chronic Disease Prevention and Health Promotion states that despite common knowledge that exercise is healthful, more than 60 percent of American adults are not regularly active, and 25 percent are not active at all. This means that only 15 percent are regularly active. These statistics are staggering. Which group do you fall into? Let's all strive to be part of the 15 percent who are regularly active.

> " Every day that you breathe is a day
> that you should work out. "
> —Pete Estabrooks

I was invited by Pete Estabrooks to attend one of his incredible TKO boxing-based sports conditioning classes. He is the owner of The Fitness Guy Gym and is the fitness editor of *Impact Magazine*. In 2015 his TKO class was voted by fitness experts to be the best workout in Calgary. I was excited to get his thoughts on what it means to be physically active—but first I had to survive one of his classes. The experts were right: it was one of the best workouts I have ever tried!

Whether you are attending his classes, reading one of his many articles or speaking with him one-on-one, one thing is clear: Pete is extremely passionate about health and fitness, and he loves to share that enthusiasm with others. Here are some of his thoughts.

> The way that you live your life between 50 and 65 will determine how you live the rest of your life. People ask me, "How often should I work out?" I say, "Every day that you breathe!" Every day that you breathe is a day that you should work out. It doesn't mean you have to be super intense all the time, but you have to do something.

> The only reason that I do fitness is so that I can really live my life, so that I can wake up every morning and can choose what I decide to do. What I want to do is completely dependent on what I have time to do, and not dependent on "Can I do that?" I'm 55. I know that how I live the next 10 years will determine how I live the next 25 years of my life.

> Some people tell me they don't have time to work out. Everybody has time to work out. If you tell yourself that you don't have time, you're lying to yourself. If you're not pursuing yourself physically in all of the aspects—strength, cardiovascular fitness and balance—then by the time you're 65, you're not living your life.

I have to admit that at 55, Pete is in phenomenal physical condition and puts most 20-year-olds to shame. Even more impressive is the fact that his mother Peggy, who is over 80, attends his TKO classes three times a week. Now that's what I call living your life!

Finding Your Why

" " The why—it focuses your energies. " "
—Michael McDonald

So what is it for you? What is your reason for getting physically active? Is it to lose weight, combat stress, keep disease at bay or feel younger? Michael McDonald, owner of Orange Theory Fitness, says that usually people walk into his fitness facility and ask, "How do I get started?" This is what he tells them.

> The question I always ask back is, "Why do you want to get started?" The why—it focuses your energies! If you're going to do this fitness thing, there has to be that meaning, that purpose, otherwise you're just doing it because you should. Then it's not going to become a habit because you're not doing it for yourself. You won't see any progress.
>
> What do you want to get out of this? What inspires you? It's different for everybody because different people have different goals. For some, it might be to get back into the community, to be around other adults. For others, it's a weight-loss goal, or an overall health goal.
>
> For a lot of women, because they've been looking after everybody else, fitness becomes that time where they reinvest in themselves. We see more and more women starting to work out in their 40s. They're trying something they've never tried before. They're changing their bodies, improving their self-esteem and their confidence.

Let's continue on the subject of the deeper why, to help you focus in on exactly what your goal is. When you say, "I want to exercise because my friend is doing it," "Because I have to," or "Because it's January 1," you will likely lack the commitment level you need in order to succeed.

I spoke with a professional life coach to find out how she would guide someone in helping her realize her deeper why and the importance of it. Daleen Pinder is a life coach who empowers women all over the country to live their best lives. This is how she helps her clients succeed.

> The importance of having a why is that it will drive you to commit to it. It will motivate you to get out of your comfort zone and push towards accomplishing your goals. The why—it's what's going to pull you through to actually getting out and exercising every day. Remind yourself daily of why this is important to you.

> I have four foundational questions that I ask in every coaching session.

>   1.   What do you truly want?
>   2.   How might you get it?
>   3.   How might you commit to that?
>   4.   How would you know if you got it?

> These questions help people become resourceful to find out what it is for them.

Rick Mueller, personal trainer at Only Women's Fitness, told me about one of his clients, Karen, and the why that keeps her coming to the gym.

> Karen suffers from arthritis, has high blood pressure and struggles with the pains of fibromyalgia. A lot of people take the ailments that they have and use them as an excuse not to exercise. But this lady is 70 years old, is incredibly fit, has a great attitude and is an example of

truly inspired and healthy living. You would never be able to tell that she has all those conditions. She has to get out to the gym. Her belief system is, "If I don't get out to the gym, these conditions are going to get worse." That's her why!

Nancy Collyer, a 50-year-old mother of three grown children, says that saying no to exercise is not an option. She guards her exercise time and makes it a priority in her schedule. In the following account, she explains her why.

I have had anemia for the last 30 years, but I just recently found out why. After having many tests done, the doctors concluded that I was born with a leaky kidney. This means that I lose blood and protein all the time in the filtration process. This causes my red blood cell count and my iron levels to plummet. I take iron supplements and greens powder to stay on top of feeling good.

But there is nothing like exercise to keep you energized. To me, exercise is a priority and goes number one in my day. I work everything else around it. Because I exercise, I find that I have a lot more energy and never get run down or sick. That's one of the hugest benefits of exercise. My doctor says to keep doing what I'm doing, because it's keeping everything at bay.

Have you thought about your personal why? I challenge you to think about it and then write down three reasons why you should make exercise a part of your day. This will help to motivate and inspire you to commit more fully to being physically active.

Five Ways to Help You Form the Exercise Habit

Now that you have established your reasons for exercising, the next step is finding ways of making exercise a habit. They say that it takes three weeks of consistently doing something in order to form a habit. All you have to do is simply begin. As Lao-tzu states, "A journey of a thousand miles begins with a single step."

Start Small

Decide today to do at least 20 minutes of exercise. It can be as simple as a walk around the park. As you experience the exhilarating feeling that follows exercise, you will look forward to increasing the intensity and duration of your physical activity.

Schedule It

Put it on a calendar, in your appointment book or as a reminder in your phone; this way it is more likely to get done. Try exercising first thing in the morning. Not only will it energize you for the day, but it will leave you with a sense of accomplishment. Get it done before the day's distractions begin.

Commit to It

Involve a friend. It is easier to stick to a program knowing that there is someone sharing that experience with you—someone counting on you to be there at the appointed time and place. You could also purchase a gym membership or enlist in an exercise class. This creates a financial commitment that may help you take the plunge into fitness.

Be Prepared

Make sure that you have every needful thing ready ahead of time. Have enough sets of workout clothes, a water bottle, a small towel and comfortable running shoes. Set these out the night before so that you are always ready to go.

Track It

Keep a record of your exercise; it will serve as a system of accountability. Record the date, the type of exercise you did, the duration, your body weight and any comments on your progress. This will help motivate you to keep going.

And remember to keep it fun!

I spoke with Cara Poppitt, a world-renowned dancer, speaker and mother of two. Her passion for fitness led her to open Soul Connexion in 2008, Calgary's only dance, yoga and fitness studio. I asked her what she would say to women who do not know where to begin in terms of exercise.

> I encourage them to find an activity they love doing, and start with a short time duration and moderate intensity. The truth is the more you enjoy doing something, the more likely you are to keep up with it and reach your goals.
>
> A lot of women tell me, "I have so many things to do. I have no time for yoga!" But when they take the time to take care of themselves and come into the studio to do a class, they begin to realize that they can be much more productive in their lives, and they feel so much better!
>
> We hear a lot of talk about depression among women. I don't know if it's because it's more prevalent, or because we are becoming more open to talking about it. So many women are saying that they feel better when they exercise. Exercise leads to the release of endorphins in the brain, which give you that natural high. So find something fun and do it!

What sorts of physical activities do you enjoy doing? When was the last time you did them? Are you engaging in exercise most days of the week?

Exercising at home is one way to stay fit. There are also many wonderful exercise classes offered at local community centres, churches and city pools.

Joining a gym is another great choice. If this is your option, I suggest you try a gym close to your home or work, making it as easy as possible to get there. Ask for a free one-week pass so you can try it out before making the financial commitment. Most gyms will charge about $35–55 a month. This fee includes the use of all gym equipment (treadmills and other cardio equipment, free weights and exercise machines). You will also be able to attend all of their group exercise classes for free. Some of the classes offered are yoga, group cycling, Zumba, strength training and a variety of fitness boot camps. For a fee, you can hire a personal trainer who will design a workout program to help you meet your goals, and who will be there to guide you as you work out.

There are many wonderful ways to increase your physical activity. Find what works best for you and make it part of your routine.

In the next section, you will learn a simple exercise routine you can use anytime and anywhere.

The Five-Minute Body-Weight Workout

Making the choice to improve your physical activity is the best thing you can do for yourself. Once you begin, you will see the many health benefits it provides. That alone should be enough to motivate you to continue to challenge yourself in new and wonderful ways.

I had the privilege of speaking with Obi Obadike, a world-renowned fitness expert and writer. He agreed that in order to improve your fitness, you don't need to purchase expensive equipment or get a gym membership, and you don't have to take hours out of your day to make it happen.

> We live in a society right now where people seem to gravitate to exercise they can do that is within reach, where

they don't have to travel too far, where they don't have to go to a gym. Walking and body-weight exercises that you can do at home seem to be attractive to the person who may not have enough time, or may not have the money to afford a gym membership.

For women over 40, I think that walking is a phenomenal cardiovascular exercise. It's accessible to everyone, and all you need is a good pair of running shoes. It's definitely a great alternative for someone who finds running too hard on their joints. Similarly, if lifting weights is too challenging on the joints, then performing low-impact body-weight exercises is a great training option for women as they get older. Exercises like jumping jacks, modified push-ups and chair dips, to name a few.

Look for Obi's new show *Sweat Inc.,* a fitness reality TV show where he co-hosts and judges alongside Jillian Michaels.

> " Movement is a medicine for creating change in a person's physical, emotional, and mental states. "
> —Carol Welch

Daily exercise shouldn't be complicated. The following workout incorporates 10 exercises you can do at home or in your travels. It requires no equipment, just your own body. The exercises encourage overall muscle strength and development, core strength, balance, flexibility and cardiovascular endurance. This workout can challenge the beginner as well as the seasoned athlete.

Begin with 5–10 minutes of low to moderate intensity cardiovascular exercise, to warm up your muscles and get your heart pumping. You can take a brisk walk, march or jog in place, walk up and down stairs or jump rope.

Each cycle of the following 10 exercises takes five minutes. Repeat the cycle four times, and you have a very efficient way of performing a 20-minute workout without having to leave home or pay for gym fees. Do this workout three days a week and include cardiovascular exercise for 30 minutes or more on alternate days, such as walking, jogging, swimming, hiking or cycling.

As you read through the explanation of the individual exercises, I invite you to take a moment to try each one so that you will become familiar with the movement. This way you will be ready for an excellent workout later on.

1. Jumping Jacks (10 repetitions)

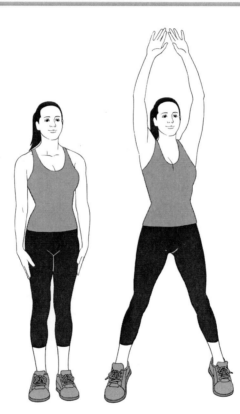

How to: Stand with your feet together and your arms by your sides. Slightly bend your knees, and make a small jump landing on your forefoot with your legs separated and your arms raised. Then jump and return to the starting position. That is one repetition. If you have difficulty jumping, you may choose to simply step out to the sides instead.

Muscles worked: This exercise stimulates blood flow to a variety of muscles in both the upper and lower body, as well as increasing your heart rate.

2. Standing Bicycle Crunches (10 repetitions per side)

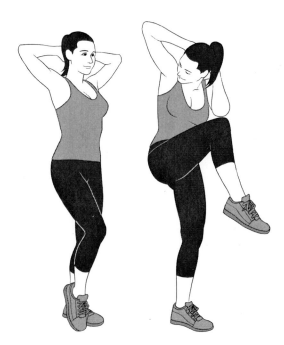

How to: Stand with your feet about hip-width apart, with your hands clasped behind your head and your elbows out to the side. Inhale and then exhale as you bend one knee and draw it up as high as you can, and bring your opposite elbow to the outside of your knee. Return to the starting position and repeat on the other side, completing a total of 20 repetitions, 10 per side. If balance is an issue, place one hand against the wall or chair and do 10 repetitions on one side, then switch sides and perform the next 10 repetitions.

Muscles worked: Abdominals (stomach muscles), obliques (sides of the stomach)

3. Reverse Lunge to Knee-up (10 repetitions per side)

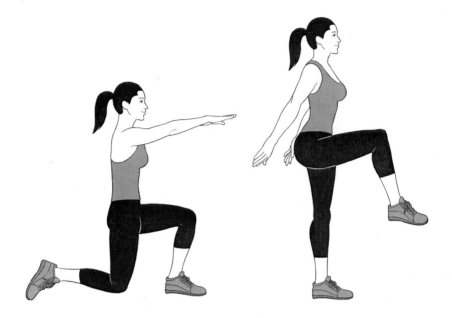

How to: Stand tall with your hands by your sides. Inhale as you take a step back and lower your knee as low as is comfortable without touching the floor. Your front leg is bent at 90 degrees with your knee directly in line with your toes. As you go down, your arms come up to the front for balance. Now exhale, push yourself up and raise your knee as far upwards as possible, keeping your back straight. Your arms move down to help propel you up. Do 10 repetitions on one side, then switch sides and perform the next 10 repetitions. If balance is an issue, place one hand against the wall or on a chair.

Muscles worked: Quadriceps (front of the leg), hamstrings (back of the leg), gluteal muscles (buttocks), calves, hip flexors (front of the hip) and lower abdominals (lower stomach region)

4. Chair Squat to Calf Raise (10 repetitions)

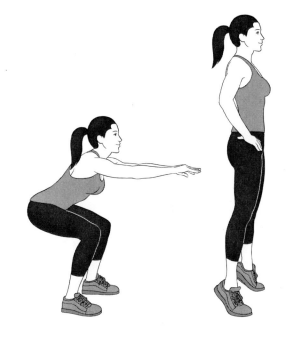

How to: With a chair behind you, stand with your feet about hip-width apart, your toes pointing forward and your arms by your sides. Tighten your abdominal muscles and look straight ahead throughout the movement. Inhale and start descending by pushing your hips back and bending your knees to lower into a squat. Keep your weight back on your heels. Stop before your buttocks come into contact with the seat of the chair. Exhale and return to the starting position, then push up onto your toes to a calf raise. Raising your arms to the front as you squat will help with balance. As you become stronger, you will perform these squats without a chair, bringing the movement down to where your thighs are parallel to the floor.

Muscles worked: Quadriceps (front of the leg), hamstrings (back of the leg), gluteal muscles (buttocks), calves, core (trunk muscles)

5. Wall Push-ups (10 repetitions)

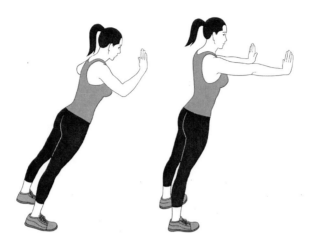

How to: Stand with your face close to the wall. Place your hands on the wall slightly wider than shoulder-width apart, and take a giant step back. You should be in the right position to begin the exercise. Inhale and bend your elbows as you lean your body towards the wall. Now exhale and push your body back, keeping your hands on the wall.

Muscles worked: Chest, shoulders, triceps (back of the arms)

6. Lying Hip Raise (10 repetitions)

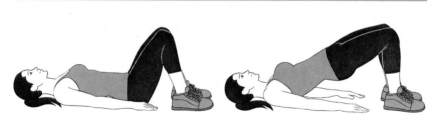

How to: Lie on your back with your knees bent, your feet on the floor and your arms by your sides with palms down. Inhale and then exhale as you raise your pelvis off the floor, squeezing your gluteal muscles (buttocks) tightly. Pause for a moment before returning to the starting position.

Muscles worked: Gluteal muscles (buttocks), hamstrings (back of the leg)

7. Triceps Floor Dips (10 repetitions)

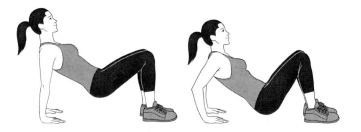

How to: Sit on the floor with your knees bent. Place your hands on the floor close to your hips, keeping your elbows bent. Take a breath, exhale and lift your hips off the floor until your arms are straight. Now inhale as you bend the elbows to lower your hips to just above the floor. Focus on straightening and bending the elbows as you repeat the exercise 10 times.

Muscles worked: Triceps (back of the arm)

8. Seated Leg Lifts (10 repetitions per side)

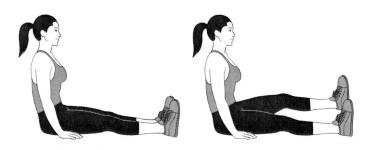

How to: Sit on the floor with your back straight and your legs extended in front of you, with your toes pointed upwards; your hands are on the floor by your hips. Now tighten the abdominal muscles and one thigh, and lift that heel off the floor. Repeat 10 times and then switch to the other leg for 10 more repetitions. This is a small movement. You may prefer to place your back against a wall for additional support.

Muscles worked: Abdominals (stomach muscles), and you will also feel the quadriceps muscles (front of the leg) being engaged

9. Kneeling Superman (10 repetitions per side)

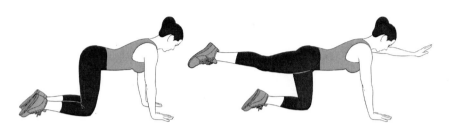

How to: Kneel on all fours, with your hands just beneath your shoulders and your knees lined up with your hips. Keeping one knee on the floor, breathe in, exhale and extend the other leg back until the heel is in line with your hips. At the same time, lift the opposite arm to shoulder level. Return to the starting position and then repeat with the opposite arm and leg. Keep your core (trunk muscles) tight to help keep your back straight. If this exercise is too difficult, extend your leg back, leaving both arms on the floor, and alternate the legs. As you get stronger, you will be able to raise the opposite arm at the same time. This is a great balance exercise.

Muscles worked: Back, gluteal muscles (buttocks), shoulders

10. Plank (hold for 10 to 30 seconds)

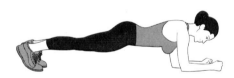

How to: Lie face down and rest your weight on your forearms, with your elbows directly below your shoulders and forming a 90-degree angle. Your knees are off the floor with just your forearms and toes for support. Keep your body in one straight line from head to ankles. Keep your core (trunk muscles) tight, and breathe. Continue to inhale and exhale as you hold to the count of 10, or longer as you become stronger. In the beginning, you may choose to modify this plank exercise by keeping your knees on the mat.

Muscles worked: Core (trunk muscles)

Full Body Stretching Routine

Flexibility is the ability to move joints through their full movement potential. Through aging, disuse, lack of stretching and poor posture, you may experience a decreased range of motion that can be accompanied by pain and injury. Regular activity and a good stretching program can help prevent loss of mobility and will significantly reduce the possibility of becoming injured or developing chronic pain.

The common belief used to be that stretching prior to the main workout was favourable. We now realize that stretching cold muscles can significantly increase your chances of a pulled or torn muscle. You can still stretch prior to training as long as you have warmed up sufficiently (5–10 minutes). But actually, the best time to stretch is after your workout, when your body is warmed up and more pliable. Working with warm muscles ensures that they will lengthen more easily and with less discomfort. An ideal post-workout stretching routine will last from 5–10 minutes.

Here are a few stretching tips to keep you fit and flexible.

How to Stretch

Stretch to the point where you feel a slight tension in the muscle. Hold that stretch gently for at least 15–30 seconds while you continue your normal breathing pattern. Stretching should never induce pain. Release your stretch for 5 seconds and then repeat the same stretch two or three times to encourage a wider range of motion at the joints. Never bounce or use a jerking motion while stretching because this can cause injury. Make sure you stretch both sides of the body equally.

Benefits of Stretching

Whether you stretch after your workout or enjoy the stretching that a yoga class provides, the long-term benefits of improved flexibility are numerous.

- Helps you perform daily activities with relative ease
- Improves athletic performance
- Improves muscle co-ordination
- Improves posture
- Improves recovery of the muscles trained
- Reduces joint degeneration
- Reduces muscle soreness and tension
- Reduces risk of developing chronic back pain
- Reduces risk of injury
- Serves as relaxation and rejuvenation for mind and body

Stretching is often overlooked, but it is an important component of a well-balanced fitness regime. Here are some stretches you can try. Make them part of your exercise routine. As you read through the explanation to the following stretches, I invite you to take a moment to practice each movement.

1. Chest/Shoulder Stretch

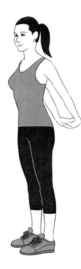

Clasp your hands behind your back. Then gently pull back with your arms, opening the chest and stretching the front of the shoulders. Hold for 15–30 seconds. Release and repeat.

2. Overhead Triceps Stretch

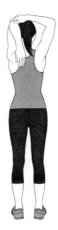

Bend your arm and reach back, placing your hand over your shoulder blade. Then grasp that elbow with the opposite hand and apply gentle pressure to pull the arm back a little. You should feel this in your triceps (back of the arm). Hold for 15–30 seconds. Release and repeat, then switch sides.

3. Arm Crossover Shoulder Stretch

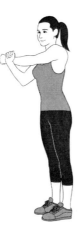

Your arm comes across your chest. Then bring the opposite arm across and place it just above your elbow. Gently pull across your body to stretch the back of the shoulder. Hold for 15–30 seconds. Release and repeat, then switch sides.

4. Standing Quadriceps Stretch

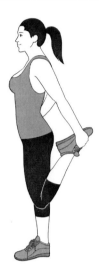

Hold on to the wall and stand on one leg. Bend the opposite leg and grab the top of your foot. Focus on keeping your knee pointing towards the floor, and create a straight line from your hip to your knee. You should feel this in your quadriceps (front of the leg). Hold for 15–30 seconds. Release and repeat, then switch sides.

5. Seated Hamstrings Stretch

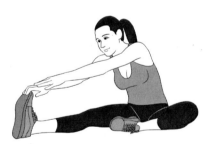

Sit on a mat with one leg extended in front of you. Bend the opposite leg and place that foot against your inner thigh. Lean forward with a nice straight back, reaching as far as is comfortable, aiming to touch your ankle or foot. You should feel a nice stretch in your hamstrings (back of the leg). Hold for 15–30 seconds. Release and repeat, then switch sides.

6. Seated Twist

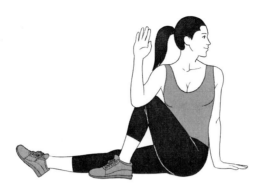

Sit tall on a mat. Bend one leg and place your foot flat on the mat. Rest your hand on the floor behind you for support. Rotate your torso, and bring the elbow of the opposite arm to the outside of your knee. Gently press the elbow into the knee to encourage your torso to twist. Release and repeat, then switch sides.

7. Lying Hip Stretch

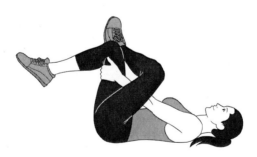

Lie on your back with one leg up and bent at 90 degrees, and the opposite leg crossed over the top. Grasp behind the knee of the bottom leg and pull it towards you as far as is comfortable. You should feel a stretch in your gluteal muscles (buttocks). Hold for 15–30 seconds. Release and repeat, then switch sides.

8. Lying Low Back Stretch

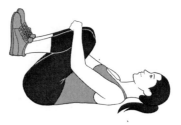

Lying on your back, hug your knees to your chest. This is a gentle stretch for your lower back. Hold for 15–30 seconds. Release and repeat.

9. Cat stretch

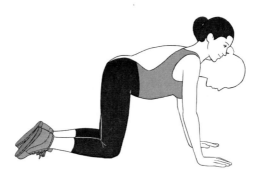

Get down on your hands and knees. Arch your back nice and high just like a cat for five seconds. Then reverse the direction and get a nice bow in your back for five seconds. Repeat. This is a gentle stretch for the entire spine.

Stay active, agile and able!

CHAPTER 5

Hormone Management

> ❝ The higher your energy level, the more efficient
> your body. The more efficient your body, the
> better you feel and the more you will use
> your talent to produce outstanding results. ❞
> —Tony Robbins

Hormonal changes happen to all women, especially after the age of 40. This is normal and part of life, but these changes can cause hormonal imbalances that can lead to physical problems. Balancing hormones is a juggling act. Hormones all work in concert, just like a juggler rotating a number of balls in the air and trying to keep them all working together.

Let's first examine the role of the adrenal glands and how important they are to your health and well-being.

The Importance of the Adrenal Glands

The adrenal glands are located on top of each kidney. Though no bigger than a walnut, these glands produce several hormones such as cortisol and adrenaline, which enable you to respond to various forms of stress. They also produce the sex hormones estrogen, progesterone, testosterone and DHEA (a precursor to the main sex hormones). All are essential for proper functioning of the body.

Here is what happens when you have low-functioning adrenal glands.

Adrenal Fatigue

A lot of people live a stressful lifestyle and suffer from adrenal fatigue without ever realizing it. This condition often goes undiagnosed. Chronic stress is one of the biggest culprits. Whether physical, mental or emotional, the adrenals work overtime during times of stress. As a woman over 40, you have all sorts of responsibilities that demand your attention in and out of the home. You might begin to feel overwhelmed and overburdened. This is when health issues can begin to develop.

If you find it difficult to get up in the morning, walk around exhausted all day and go to bed worn out, you could be suffering from adrenal fatigue. Besides being constantly tired, other symptoms of adrenal fatigue are:

- Anxiety and depression
- Brain fog
- Cravings for sugar
- Difficulty sleeping
- Diminished sex drive
- Hot flashes
- Low thyroid function and low blood pressure
- Weight gain and poor digestion

Testing Your Adrenal Glands at Home

Here is a quick and easy way to check if your adrenal glands are functioning properly. This test requires the use of a home blood-pressure monitor.

- Lie down for five minutes. Take your blood pressure in this horizontal position. Make note of the top number (systolic pressure).
- After five minutes, stand up and take your blood pressure again.

With healthy adrenal function, you should see an increase in the systolic pressure of about 10 mm Hg from lying to standing. If instead the top number drops by 10 mm Hg, you have poor-functioning adrenal glands and may be struggling with adrenal fatigue. If it drops by more than 10 mm Hg, you have adrenal exhaustion.

How to Restore Adrenal Health

Adrenal health can be restored through proper nutrition and supplementation, as well as implementing stress reduction techniques. Follow these guidelines.

- Eat nutritious meals and snacks at regular intervals, every three to four hours. Each meal should contain protein, complex carbohydrates and healthy fats for sustained energy. Ensure that you include plenty of fresh fruits and vegetables.

- Begin your day with breakfast no later than one hour after rising. Have a mid-morning snack followed by lunch, a mid-afternoon snack, dinner and a light snack an hour before bed (if desired). This bedtime snack may help avoid sleep disturbances. Spacing meals in this manner will keep your energy levels balanced throughout the day. This also prevents blood sugar from dropping, which causes cortisol to be released as the body perceives a stressful situation.

- Increase your intake of vitamin C foods such as bell peppers, berries, citrus fruits and dark leafy greens. You can also take a vitamin C supplement during especially stressful times.

- B complex vitamins help support the proper function of the adrenal glands. A diet of whole foods will ensure that you have an adequate intake of this group of vitamins. Dark leafy greens, eggs, grains, salmon, chicken, beans and lentils, and nuts and seeds are great B complex foods. A supplement may also be required if you struggle with adrenal fatigue. Check with your doctor.

- Limit the following foods: sugar, caffeinated drinks, chocolate, alcohol and nicotine. These cause the adrenal glands to work harder, leading to exhaustion.

- Adopt tools and activities to help reduce your stress on a daily basis. See chapter 7 for some stress-reduction techniques.

- Don't over-exercise. Exercising for longer than 60 consecutive minutes will tax your adrenals.

- Remember the importance of adequate sleep; at least seven to eight hours a night. See chapter 6 for tips to help you sleep better.

You may be wondering how long it takes to restore adrenal health. This depends on how long you have been struggling with fatigue. By following these nutrition and lifestyle suggestions, it is conceivable to recover within six months. For those who have been suffering for years, this would take considerably longer, up to two years of consistently following these recommendations.

The Importance of the Thyroid Gland

The thyroid gland, a butterfly-shaped gland along the front of the neck, is critical to many functions. The hormones it produces regulate body temperature, metabolism, growth and development, heart rate and blood pressure.

Thyroid Problems

The most common thyroid problem is hypothyroidism, otherwise known as underactive thyroid. This is when your thyroid does not make enough thyroid hormones. This slows down many of your body's functions, such as your metabolism. This is more prevalent in women than in men.

Here is a brief quiz taken from the Nutri-Body assessment method created by Professor David W. Rowland. These conditions, and many others, can be associated with hypothyroidism. Check the statements that apply to you.

( ) Fail to feel rested, even after sleeping long hours
( ) Start slow in the morning, gain speed in the afternoon
( ) Cold hands or feet
( ) Sensitivity to cold; prefer warm climate
( ) Hair scanty, dry, brittle, dull, lustreless, lifeless
( ) Flaky, dry, rough skin
( ) Sleeplessness, restlessness, sleep disturbances
( ) Constipation, less than one bowel movement daily
( ) Diminished sex drive, lack of sexual desire
( ) Gain weight easily, fail to lose on diets
( ) Poor short-term memory, forgetfulness
( ) Irritability, mood swings
( ) Multiple food allergies/sensitivities
( ) Depression

If you have checked three or more of these statements, you may be struggling with an underactive thyroid.

Testing Your Thyroid at Home

In addition to taking this quiz, you can check your temperature to assess the function of your thyroid. Taking a basal temperature test is an effective way of determining if you have an underactive thyroid. This method was developed almost 60 years ago by Dr. Broda Barnes.

- Shake down a liquid-type (mercury) thermometer and place it by your bedside.

- Upon awakening and before stirring from bed, place the bulb of the thermometer under your armpit and hold it there for 10 minutes.

- Record the reading on two consecutive days. A range of 36.6–36.8°C (97.8– 98.2°F) suggests normal thyroid function. Temperatures below 36.6°C (97.8°F) indicate low thyroid function.

  Menstruating women should do this test on the second and third mornings after their flow starts in order to eliminate temperature fluctuations that accompany one's cycle. Post-menopausal women can take this test at any time.

Alternatively, you can take oral temperature readings with a mercury thermometer between the hours of 10:00 a.m. and 5:00 p.m. This method is suggested by Professor David W. Rowland in his book the *Vitamost Encyclopedia of Food Based Medicines*.

- Take at least four oral temperature readings between the hours of 10:00 a.m. and 5:00 p.m. Use an old-fashioned mercury thermometer for this type of testing; it is more accurate than a digital thermometer.

- Calculate the average. To paint a more accurate picture, use the average of readings taken over several days. For this test, an average temperature below 37°C (98.6°F) suggests a low-functioning thyroid.

How to Restore Thyroid Health

A comprehensive approach to correcting poor thyroid function must also provide support to the adrenal glands. Often the thyroid goes low because the adrenal glands are overworked. It is a conserving mechanism. Therefore following the guidelines for adrenal health is a good place to begin. Here are some additional dietary suggestions.

Iodine and selenium are the two most important minerals required for optimal thyroid function. The following are some foods that are high in these minerals.

- **Iodine:** Dried sea vegetables such as kelp, nori, wakame and dulse are high in iodine and add a salty taste to foods. These can be used in soups, salads and sushi. Kelp is also available in capsule form at your local health food store as well as in granule form, which you can sprinkle on salads and other dishes.

- **Selenium:** Seafood such as shrimp and oysters are high in selenium. Other foods high in selenium include brazil nuts, sunflower and chia seeds, mushrooms, brown rice, quinoa, lima and pinto beans, and leafy green vegetables.

Here are other beneficial nutrients that support the thyroid.

- **Omega-3 fatty acids:** Include fatty fish such as salmon and sardines, flax seed oil, and nuts and seeds such as almonds, pecans, walnuts, ground flax seeds, chia seeds and pumpkin seeds in your daily diet.

- **Vitamin A:** Carrots and sweet potatoes are excellent, plant-based sources of vitamin A.

- **Vitamin D:** It can be taken in supplement form; check with your doctor for dosage. You can also drink beverages that are fortified with vitamin D.

- **Zinc:** Pumpkin seeds and sesame seeds are great sources of zinc.

Adding foods to your diet that are rich in the above nutrients can help improve your nutrition and give your body the building blocks it needs for making the thyroid hormones.

It is also important to limit certain foods that are high in goitrogens. Goitrogens are substances that suppress thyroid function by interfering with iodine absorption. Leafy greens such as bok choi, broccoli, Brussels sprouts, cabbage and kale should be steamed to reduce the goitrogens. Also reduce the amount of soy in your diet for the same reason.

In addition to a nutrient-dense diet, daily exercise and stress management can be very beneficial if you are struggling with an underactive thyroid. See chapter 4 and chapter 7 for additional help.

Balancing the Sex Hormones

Estrogen, progesterone and testosterone are the three sex hormones, with estrogen and progesterone being more dominant in females. They need to function in balance to maintain optimal health. Estrogen, produced by the ovaries, helps develop and maintain female characteristics. Progesterone controls menstruation and helps prepare for pregnancy. Testosterone is produced in smaller amounts in females; it helps with bone health and maintaining muscle.

What Happens When Hormone Levels Drop?

As a woman moves closer to menopause, she enters a period called perimenopause. It can begin as early as 10 years before complete cessation of menstruation. It is a time when the ovaries gradually produce less and less estrogen and progesterone. Periods become irregular. The flow could be lighter or even heavier.

After a year with no menstrual cycles, a woman enters menopause; her childbearing years are over. The ovaries cease to produce estrogen and progesterone, and that job is now taken over primarily by the adrenal glands. Therefore it becomes even more vital to maintain adrenal health.

As hormone levels start to drop and the body seeks to re-establish balance, certain symptoms attributed to menopause begin to emerge. Here is a list of menopausal symptoms experienced by women with some tips you can use to help improve the conditions.

- **Hot Flashes**
    - Avoid hot temperatures
    - Avoid spicy foods, alcohol and caffeine
    - Dress in layers

- Drink ice cold water
- Keep a hot flash journal to observe possible triggers
- Participate in physical activities that will increase your cardiovascular health
- Use cotton sheets and cotton sleepwear
- Use stress-management techniques
- Wear natural fabrics

- **Lack of Focus**
  - Adopt better sleep habits
  - Eat a healthy diet that includes omega-3 fatty acids
  - Stay active
  - Use stress-management techniques

- **Mood Swings**
  - Limit caffeine and sugar
  - Eat smaller meals more often
  - Exercise in the great outdoors

- **Osteoporosis**
  - Limit alcohol; it interferes with calcium absorption
  - Limit caffeine from beverages such as coffee, tea and cola; caffeine increases the amount of calcium excreted in urine
  - Limit salt (sodium); it increases the amount of calcium excreted in urine
  - Stop smoking; it decreases calcium absorption
  - Eat a healthy, balanced diet rich in fruits and vegetables, protein, healthy fats and fibre
  - Eat calcium-rich foods: broccoli, kale, collard greens and other leafy green vegetables, as well as canned salmon and sardines with bones, almonds and dairy
  - Take calcium and vitamin D supplements; check with your doctor for requirement and dosage
  - Do regular weight-bearing exercise to help strengthen the bones

- **Poor Sleep**
  - Avoid caffeine later in the day
  - Keep the bedroom cool
  - Maintain a regular sleep schedule

  See chapter 6 for additional help.

- **Urinary Problems**
  - Eat foods high in vitamin C: dark leafy greens and citrus fruits; they support healthy collagen production, which helps maintain urinary tract elasticity to prevent leakages
  - Consult a physiotherapist who specializes in pelvic health
  - Do Kegel exercises to strengthen the pelvic floor. Squeeze the same muscles that you would use to stop the flow of urine. Hold for 3 seconds and then relax. Repeat 10–15 times. Gradually build up to holding a squeeze for 10 seconds. This exercise can be done while you are lying down, sitting or standing.

- **Vaginal Dryness**
  - Eat foods high in vitamin C: dark leafy greens and citrus fruits; they support healthy collagen production, which helps treat vaginal dryness
  - Include more vitamin E foods: almonds, sunflower seeds, avocados and dark leafy greens
  - Increase your intake of omega-3 fatty acids
  - Use organic, water-based lubricants free of parabens

- **Weight Gain**

  Excessive fat tissue produces more estrogen. Therefore it is important to maintain a healthy weight to help keep the hormone system balanced.
  - Eat a healthy diet low in sugary treats and other simple carbohydrates such as white flour
  - Enjoy six smaller meals a day to improve your metabolism
  - Space your meals three to four hours apart to maintain healthy blood sugar levels

- Incorporate more physical activity into your day
- Lift weights

Symptoms of Estrogen Dominance

When your body's sex hormones aren't working in concert, symptoms of estrogen dominance will arise. You can have low, normal or excessive estrogen with little or no progesterone to balance its effects in the body. Therefore, even with low estrogen levels, you can experience symptoms of estrogen dominance if you don't have enough progesterone.

Here is a list of some of the common symptoms experienced by women with estrogen dominance.

- Decreased sex drive
- Endometriosis
- Fat gain around the middle
- Magnesium deficiency
- Memory loss
- Mood disorders such as depression and anxiety
- Osteoporosis
- PMS and irregular and heavy periods
- Polycystic ovaries
- Swelling and tenderness in the breasts
- Thyroid dysfunction, cold hands and feet, fatigue
- Uterine fibroids
- Water retention and bloating

Hormone Disruptors That Cause Estrogen Dominance

Menopause is a natural event in a woman's life that can cause a hormonal imbalance, but there are other harmful things in your everyday life that are hormone disruptors. These hormone disruptors are estrogens that are not produced in your body but come from your environment. These substances are called xenoestrogens—chemical compounds that mimic estrogen and can cause a hormone imbalance in a woman's body.

The balance between estrogen and progesterone is vital to maintaining optimal health. Xenoestrogens can cause an estrogen to progesterone imbalance resulting in estrogen dominance. Being exposed to these chemical compounds, even to a small degree, can cause them to build up in your system. This will eventually damage your health.

It is difficult to avoid all environmental toxins and hormone disrupting chemicals because they are readily found in everyday items in our homes and places of work—in carpets, paint, furniture, food, beauty products and more. Here are some things you can do to minimize your exposure to harmful chemicals that can cause a hormonal imbalance.

- **Growth hormones and antibiotics:** Commercially raised animals are given growth hormones, antibiotics and other drugs that are passed on to humans. Choose meats and other animal products that have been raised organically without the use of hormones, antibiotics or other drugs.

- **Industrial chemicals:** These are found in personal care products, cleaning products, household pesticides and much more. They can enter your body through the skin and via inhalation. Choose products containing natural ingredients.

- **Pesticides and herbicides:** These are found on commercially produced fruits and vegetables. Purchase organic produce as much as possible. Consult ewg.org for their "Shopper's Guide to Pesticides in Produce."

- **Petrochemical compounds:** These are found in soaps, lotions, shampoos, perfumes and hairspray. Choose natural personal care products free of chemical compounds derived from petroleum.

- **Plastics:** A harmful compound called BPA (Bisphenol A) is used in the production of plastics. Avoid heating or storing foods in plastic wrap or plastic containers. Use glass instead.

- **Preservatives:** BHA and BHT are preservatives used in cosmetics and personal care products such as lipsticks and lotions. Choose natural products. They are also widely used to preserve food products such as breakfast cereal. Check the food label to make sure the product you are purchasing does not contain these preservatives.

Dietary Changes to Improve Hormone Balance

In chapter 3, you have already learned that proper nutrition is very important to hormone balance. Earlier in this chapter, you also learned that excessive fat tissue creates a hormone imbalance by producing more estrogen. Therefore controlling your weight is also key to hormone balance.

In addition to eating well and managing your weight, follow these important dietary guidelines to help you achieve hormone balance.

- To help maintain adrenal health, avoid foods with added sugar, and limit the use of alcohol, energy drinks, caffeinated teas, and coffee. More than two 8 ounce cups of brewed coffee can affect estrogen levels, increasing the uncomfortable symptoms of menopause such as hot flashes, night sweats, anxiety and irritability. Switch to caffeine-free herbal tea such as peppermint or ginger tea.

- Avoid processed soy products because they can lead to an estrogen imbalance. These are often found in processed and packaged foods. Instead, consume organic, fermented soy products such as miso and tempeh in moderation.

- Limit your consumption of high-fat red meat and high-fat dairy, because most hormone disrupting chemicals are found in fat cells.

- Consume foods that are rich in healthy, hormone-balancing fats: avocados, nuts and seeds and their butters, fatty fish such as salmon and sardines, and oils such as coconut oil, flax seed oil and olive oil.

- Eat cruciferous vegetables to help balance estrogen levels: broccoli, Brussels sprouts, cabbage, cauliflower and kale. Steam them if you have thyroid issues.

- Eat fibre-rich foods: fruits and vegetables, beans and lentils, grains, flax and chia seeds. Fibre is necessary to help flush out excess estrogen.

- Purchase organic fruits and vegetables as much as possible to reduce your exposure to hormone disrupting pesticides and herbicides. See chapter 2 for a list of fruits and vegetables with the lowest pesticide load.

- Purchase organic meat, eggs and dairy to help minimize your exposure to hormones, antibiotics and other drugs used in animals.

Herbal Remedies

For centuries women have been turning to herbs to help alleviate menopausal symptoms. There are many plants that have been used by generations of women. Here is a list of some of the plants commonly used to support healthy estrogen levels and to help quell menopausal symptoms:

- Ashwagandha: helps reduce hot flashes, anxiety and other mood disorders
- Black cohosh: used as an alternative to hormone replacement therapy
- Chasteberry: helps reduce hot flashes, night sweats, vaginal dryness and mild depression
- Passionflower: improves depression
- Red clover: helps reduce hot flashes
- Sage: helps reduce hot flashes and night sweats
- Wild yam: used as an alternative to hormone replacement therapy

Natural therapies require patience. Keep track of your progress over a trial period. Also keep in mind that no two women will be alike in what works best for them.

There are herbal remedies that combine various supportive herbs. This may be more beneficial in minimizing the symptoms than a single herb. Herbal products are safe and effective, but it is always best to consult with your doctor, especially if you are taking medications.

If you are experiencing a chronic case of any of the hormone imbalance symptoms listed in this section, then you may need to talk to your doctor about possible solutions. This is illustrated in the following story. Lynsay eventually found a medical doctor who also practiced as a naturopathic doctor. Following his advice, she was able to balance her hormones and regain her health.

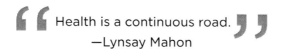

> Health is a continuous road.
> —Lynsay Mahon

Lynsay Mahon's health changed dramatically due to a prolonged period of extreme stress for her and her family. It affected her hormones, depleted her energy, increased her weight and made her severely deficient in many health-giving vitamins and minerals.

> Suddenly, four years ago I started to put on weight. It was hormonal, I was sure. The family and I went through some tough times; we had a traumatic event come into our lives, and stress levels were through the roof. Unfortunately, levels of stress maintained at that height for three years had a negative effect on my health. It was really difficult to heal during that time.
>
> Despite the fact that I was eating really well, I put on 20 pounds. It's been tough for me because I just want to lose it. I just want the weight to come off, but my body has different plans.

Lynsay found out that she had Hashimoto's disease. Hashimoto's is an autoimmune disease that affects the thyroid. The immune system mistakenly attacks and damages the thyroid, resulting in hypothyroidism. Some of the accompanying symptoms are extreme fatigue, weight gain, joint and muscle pain and digestive problems.

Hashimoto's slowed down everything. It wasn't just the weight gain, but low energy levels too. My adrenals were low as well. Normally I would be able to go a hundred miles an hour all day long. But now, I had only a good six hours in my day. At about two o'clock my energy would run out. Then by eight o'clock I was done. I really had to be great with time management. I had to recognize that it wasn't possible to work out at six o'clock at night. I needed to get my workout done earlier in the day.

I also developed many problems with food digestion. It seemed like everything I was eating caused problems: bloating, really upset stomach, never feeling great. I also started developing rheumatoid arthritis in my hands and feet.

I was tired of being tired all the time. I said, "This can't continue!" Through some research, I found something called the autoimmune protocol, which is an elimination diet. I started practising that about two years ago. It's a grain-free, dairy-free, soy-free, egg-free, nut-free diet, and you really limit the nightshade vegetables (potatoes, tomatoes, peppers and eggplant). I also had zero sugar— none. I was strict with that for a year. I would say that I saw some improvement with the digestion. Through all that, I was still not losing weight.

At that time I was also trying to investigate whether the medical community could help me. In the end, I found a medical doctor who practices as a naturopath. I have had better results in the past six months than I have had in four years. He ran an entire panel of tests. We discovered that I was absolutely depleted in vitamins A, D and E, so we have been supplementing that. When you have somebody who has digestive issues in the small intestine, you have absorption issues.

[Note: The small intestine is where fat-soluble vitamins A, D, E and K are absorbed. See chapter 3 for ways to improve your digestion.]

We also discovered that it was not just the thyroid hormone that I was lacking (for which I am taking desiccated thyroid)—it was many. I was bottomed out in DHEA hormone, so we started supplementing that. I would say that's made the biggest difference so far. I'm starting to feel like a human again. He also started supplementing progesterone. I was estrogen dominant because there was not enough progesterone to balance things out. I had been getting what felt like a mini stroke. My vision would go tunnel vision, and I would feel terrible. It was a rush of anxiety in my chest and would last anywhere from 20 seconds to a minute. I could not function while it was happening. He said that I was actually having an atypical migraine that can often be triggered by an estrogen imbalance. That is when he started me on progesterone. And ever since he started me on that, it has gone away.

Another thing that has gone away is the rheumatoid arthritis in my hands and feet. Earlier this year, my naturopath did an allergy panel with me. I have never had allergies tested; I just went with an elimination diet—the autoimmune protocol. He ran a panel of 96 foods. It came back that the only things that were off the chart were all beans (including green beans) and avocado, which was something that I was eating almost every day. I took those out of my diet, and suddenly all of the allergy symptoms went away. I've been able to reintroduce dairy and eggs, which has been like the heavens opening up for me. I still don't do great with grains. I've also reintroduced some nightshade vegetables. I have flexibility in my diet again, and it has been a big relief.

I began to feel better. My energy was better too, the rheumatoid arthritis in my hands and feet was gone and my digestion had improved. But I still needed to deal with the extra weight.

I found a really excellent personal trainer who tried to get me to refocus. Instead of focusing on weight loss, she looked at me and said, "Lynsay, you don't need to lose weight. You are a fit, beautiful person. What you're going to do instead is focus on weight training. You have that body type where you are meant to be muscular."

She started me on heavy lifting. For the past eight weeks I have been lifting heavy weights, and I love it! I finally lost five pounds. I am also starting to see positive changes in my shoulders and my arms, and I'm feeling great! It empowers you.

I will be 40 in a few weeks. One of the things that's on my mind as I approach 40 is menopause. I know it's around the corner, and what's going to happen to my hormones then?

Health is a long-term vision for sure. It's important for me to realize that it is a journey, and it is not finished. Even though I'm feeling really good right now, there is still a lot of work to do. Health is a continuous road.

More and more women today find that dealing with menopausal symptoms is best accomplished with a combination of following a healthy lifestyle and alternative treatments. It is important to note that although alternative treatments such as herbs and acupuncture do work for many women, there are situations where advice from your doctor is warranted.

CHAPTER 6

Sleep Management

> " Health is the first muse, and sleep
> is the condition to produce it. "
> —Ralph Waldo Emerson

We often overlook sleep as an important factor in our health and well-being. We may be adopting healthier eating habits and going to the gym a few times a week, but do we really take our sleep seriously?

Lack of proper sleep is quite prevalent in today's society, especially among women in midlife. Sleep disturbances are common as women transition into menopause. Symptoms such as night sweats can significantly decrease a woman's quality of sleep. Add to that all the pressures, worries, people needing our care and the long lists of things to do, it is no wonder that our health is suffering. We can't sleep, we lack focus, we feel depressed, we struggle with our weight and we open ourselves up to the risk of disease.

We all need the restorative benefits of sleep. Sleep helps us repair, renew and feel energized. It relaxes our body and rests our mind so we can perform better the next day. Sleep improves our mood and mental health. It strengthens our immune system making us less prone to catching colds and the flu. And as we will learn later in this chapter, sleep also helps us manage our weight.

Remember when you used to get 12 hours of uninterrupted sleep as a teenager, and now you can barely sleep five solid hours? You know that you should get seven to eight hours of sleep a night—you've been told this for years. As you lie awake thinking about that project at work, worrying about your teenage son, or lying there soaked in sweat, sleep deprivation is robbing you of your health and vitality. It is time to get serious about reclaiming your beauty sleep!

Establish a Good Sleep Routine

> " Sleep is that golden chain that ties
> health and our bodies together. "
> —Thomas Dekker

Don't you wish you could press a switch and immediately fall into peaceful, restful slumber? Keep in mind that good sleep begins long before your head hits the pillow.

Bedtime Rituals

- **Unplug:** An hour before bed, you should stop using your electronic devices: the television, the computer, your laptop, your phone and other technology. The bright lights and the distraction are too stimulating as you are trying to wind down. And remember, technology should never be part of your bedroom. Your bedroom is for two things only: rest and relationships.

- **Relax before bed**: This could be having a cup of tea, listening to quiet music, curling up with a good book, having an Epsom salts bath, writing in your gratitude journal, praying, or meditating. All these activities are conducive to relaxation and will prepare you for slumber.

- **Keep a consistent bedtime:** Getting to bed at a regular time most nights of the week will increase your chances of falling asleep and staying asleep. Your body will be programmed to start winding down at a certain time.

Your Bedroom

- **Keep it cool:**

  - Have a cool shower before bed.
  - Keep the bedroom temperature at a slightly lower temperature than would be comfortable during the day. This makes you feel cozy, which helps induce sleep. Use a fan or air conditioner in the hotter months, and turn down the thermostat before bed in the colder months.
  - Adopt cotton sheets with a thread count of no higher than 400. This looser weave breathes better. Also wash your sheets often, every week to 10 days, for a fresher feel as you sleep.
  - Have a wet cloth by your bedside to help cool you down.
  - Wear loose-fitting cotton sleepwear.

- **Keep it dark:** Invest in curtains or blinds that keep light out. Think of your bedroom as a cool, dark cave. Another good way to keep the light out is to wear a sleep mask.

- **Keep it quiet:** Some people prefer some white noise to help them fall asleep. Others prefer complete silence. Invest in a pair of ear plugs to achieve this, especially if you have a snoring partner.

- **Relaxing scents:** A few drops of lavender essential oil on your pillow will help you relax.

- **Be good to your back:** When sleeping on your back, place a small pillow under your knees to help maintain the natural curve of your lower back. This will help tense muscles to relax. Transfer that pillow to between your knees when sleeping on your side. Also, make sure you have a good pillow that will support your neck, and that your mattress is comfortable.

Things to Keep in Mind

- **Avoid daytime naps**: Although naps are deemed healthy, if you are having sleep problems, you should try to steer away from daytime napping. This can rob you of important nighttime sleep. Go to bed early instead.

- **Don't exercise too close to bedtime:** Stretching or gentle yoga is great as a way to help calm your body and mind before sleep. But other forms of vigorous exercise should be done at least two hours prior to your scheduled bedtime, to give your body a chance to wind down. Exercising in the morning is ideal because it gets your day off to an energetic start.

Dietary Cautions

- **Alcohol:** If you drink alcohol in the evening, have it at least three hours prior to bedtime. Alcohol too close to bedtime will rob you of deep, restorative sleep (REM sleep). It also dilates the blood vessels, causing a warming sensation that can spark night sweats. Opt instead for a soothing cup of herbal tea such as chamomile or lemon balm. If desired, you may refrigerate the tea so you can experience both a cooling and a calming effect.

- **Caffeine:** If you are a coffee drinker, have your last cup no later than early afternoon. Ideally, you should replace your coffee with caffeine-free herbal tea.

- **Smoking:** Nicotine is a stimulant, and smoking before bed can keep you wide awake. Consider quitting.

- **Spicy foods**: Avoid spicy foods at dinner; these have a tendency of raising your core temperature.

- **Never eat a heavy meal before bed**: First of all, this promotes fat storage because you will not be utilizing this fuel during sleep.

It also encourages acid reflux if you lie down with an undigested meal in your stomach. In addition, because your body is busy digesting this heavy meal, you will likely experience a restless night.

Eating well-balanced meals during the day will help you avoid overeating at dinner time. Eat your dinner two to three hours before your bedtime; this way your stomach has time to digest the meal.

- **Light bedtime snack:** If you do feel hungry after dinner, have a small snack an hour before bed. Usually eating something that is no more than 150 calories is best. Eat just enough food so that you can sleep and not wake up in the middle of the night feeling hungry. Focus on a snack containing protein and fat—for example, half a cup of Greek yogurt sprinkled with some nuts or seeds.

- **Avoid eating grains and sugar after dinner:** Grains and sugary foods will raise your blood sugar and prevent you from falling asleep. Then as your blood sugar drops later in the night, it will trigger a stress response in your body. This increases levels of cortisol and adrenaline, which could wake you up, and you may not be able to fall asleep again.

Addressing Common Sleep Problems

> If you can't sleep, then get up and do something instead of lying there worrying. It's the worry that gets you, not the lack of sleep.
> —Dale Carnegie

We have addressed some ways to help you get to sleep. But what happens if you wake during the night and can't get back to sleep?

Helpful Tips

- **Stay in bed for 15 minutes:** Give yourself a chance to get back to sleep. Try the meditation for beginners that you will learn about in chapter 7 on stress management.
  Focus on your breathing and on repeating a specific word or phrase over and over again. This will shift your focus away from the fact that you can't sleep, and it will slow your breathing to relax your whole body.

- **Get out of bed:** If you have not been successful in re-establishing sleep within 15 minutes, you need to get out of bed and go into another room. You don't want to associate the bedroom with stress and sleep problems. Read something that will not excite your senses. Listen to quiet music. Take notes and make to-do lists of things that may be keeping you awake. Write in your journal, but remember to keep the lights dim. Don't turn on your electronic devices; the bright lights and the sensory overload will destroy any chance you may have had of getting back to sleep.

- **Going back to bed:** Don't return to bed until your body feels ready for bed again. Once you start to feel sleepy, go back to your bed.

Holistic Help

Here are some holistic measures you can take to help you achieve restorative sleep.

- **Acupuncture:** Traditional Chinese acupuncture focuses on treating the root of the imbalance that is causing the sleep issues.

- **Aromatherapy:** Filling your surroundings with pleasant, natural scents can be very relaxing. Lavender is an essential oil that is commonly used to induce relaxation.

- **Deep breathing:** Take a deep breath that fills your abdomen. Hold this for a few seconds and then release. Focus on this simple action.

- **Epsom salts bath:** Epsom salts are magnesium sulphate mineral salts that encourage relaxation. Stir a cup of salts into your nighttime bath.

- **Herbal tea:** Chamomile and lemon balm tea calm the nervous system; this helps with sleeplessness and anxiety.

- **Massage:** A relaxing massage is a natural, drug-free way to help you sleep better, especially if your sleep problems are related to stress or pain.

- **Meditation:** Focus on your breath, and repeat a word or phrase (a mantra).

- **Yoga:** Certain yoga poses and stretches can help you unwind. They relax both body and mind to help you prepare for sleep.

Jo Yee tells of how acupuncture helped her regain restorative sleep. She had gone for 12 years without having a full night's sleep. She met with different doctors, but none were able to help her. She finally went back to her roots and what she had been taught as a child.

> Twelve years ago, I was sick. I had a cold that would not go away. I struggled with it for months. I couldn't sleep well most of the time. This unbalanced my system and started to create emotional problems as well. I developed anxiety and panic attacks. This started a vicious cycle. The less I slept, the more anxious I became.

> I am now in my early 40s, and for the first time in a very long time, I am sleeping eight consecutive hours.

It was my aunt who finally told me that I should try what had worked for our people for centuries: acupuncture. The acupuncturist explained that it would take about six treatments before I experienced results. By the third treatment, I was already sleeping a full eight hours.

I am so grateful. I feel revitalized and able to focus at work. And best of all, the anxiety and panic attacks are gone!

Sleep is so essential to your well-being. If you are having problems sleeping or staying asleep, try a combination of the suggestions in this chapter to find what works best for you, so you too can enjoy a full night of restful and restorative sleep.

Sleep and the Weight Connection

> For weight management, sleep is as important as diet and exercise.
> —Dr. Mike Bracko

So many women struggle with their weight starting in their 40s. The reasons are varied, including hormonal changes, stress, poor nutrition or lack of exercise. What about the lack of sleep? How does it affect weight gain? When I spoke with Dr. Mike Bracko, he explained the association between reduced sleep and weight gain in women over 40.

This is the number one thing women over 40 should be concerned about if they don't get enough hours of sleep or the proper quality of sleep. The easiest way to describe what happens is there is a switching on and a switching off of hormones. There is a switching off of the hormone that tells our brain that we are full (leptin hormone)— in other words, that we have eaten the amount of food where we feel satisfied. It turns that off, and then it turns on the hormone that tells us to eat, and primarily to eat high-fat foods (ghrelin hormone). We have a tendency to want to eat more, yet we don't feel satisfied. Then you're in danger of the middle-age spread.

This, in combination with the difference in hormone levels as you go into perimenopause, can certainly adversely affect your health. In addition, lack of sleep produces more cortisol. Cortisol is implicated in so many things, in particular increased storage of fat, especially belly fat. Not to mention that lack of sleep also affects cognitive function and enhances feelings of anxiety and depression.

Adding to what Dr. Bracko expressed, when you have not had enough sleep, it contributes to weight gain in other ways as well. You will feel too tired to exercise—something that is essential to help keep your weight under control. Also, when your energies are low, it will be far easier to reach for comfort foods and ready-to-eat snacks rather than cook a healthy meal. It seems fair to conclude that the less you sleep, the more likely you are to gain weight.

Examine your sleep habits and some of the problems you may be experiencing. Review the suggestions made in this chapter to help improve your daily sleep. Decide today to try at least one of the ideas in this chapter. If you wish to experiment with deep breathing and meditation, there are easy-to-follow instructions provided in the next chapter.

> " True silence is the rest of the mind, and is to the spirit what sleep is to the body— nourishment and refreshment. "
> —William Penn

CHAPTER 7

Stress Management

Are you experiencing headaches? Are you feeling tired all the time? Do you suffer from bouts of depression? You are not alone. Like many women over 40, you are probably experiencing the ill effects of stress. At this stage of your life, you may be facing numerous responsibilities and tasks, and your health could be taking a back seat. Perhaps you are taking care of children or even grandchildren. Maybe it is a career that keeps you busy. For some, it could be caring for aging parents. In addition to all of this, you may be dealing with hormonal changes. Allowing your body to take in all of these obligations, worries and pressures that you cannot possibly control or deal with all by yourself can take quite a toll on your health.

In today's busy society, people seem to accept stress as part of daily life. Some even seem to thrive on it. However, no matter how you look at it, the rigours of stress can damage your health.

Common Symptoms of Stress

Your body has ways of showing stress, and it is important to be aware of them. It will send you signs in hopes that you will pay attention and take action. It is essential to catch these initial indications of stress as early as possible, before they develop into problems that can have serious consequences.

If you experience one or more of the following symptoms on a regular basis, it is time to take stock of your life and make some adjustments before conditions become chronic. If any of these symptoms are acute, you should consult your doctor.

- Back, neck and shoulder pain
- Chronic fatigue
- Depression and anxiety
- Difficulty falling asleep
- Digestive issues
- Frequent colds, and flu
- Headaches
- Irritability
- Jaw clenching, or teeth grinding
- Rapid heartbeat
- Weight fluctuation

The Effects of Stress on Your Body

Our response to stressors—what is called the fight-or-flight response—is in fact quite natural and necessary to our survival and success as a human race. Regulated by our sympathetic nervous system, this is an automatic response that prepares us for action when a threat is perceived.

Let's examine what happens on a physiological level to a body under stress. We will use the example of a primitive woman meeting a sabre tooth tiger. When primitive woman faced this deadly predator, all of her bodily resources were activated to give her energy for immediate action—to either fight the animal or flee.

In response to the stressor, her adrenal glands secreted the stress hormones adrenaline and cortisol. Cortisol ensured that there was a steady supply of blood sugar for energy by mobilizing stored glucose (sugar) from the liver. Adrenaline raised her blood pressure, heart rate and breathing rate to assist her in dealing with the immediate danger. Blood flow to her limbs and muscles was increased, being diverted from bodily functions deemed unnecessary in the moment, such as digestion, immunity, growth and the reproductive drive.

Once the danger had passed and primitive woman had dealt with the predator by either killing it or successfully escaping from danger, she returned to a state of calm and balance within a short time. We call this the rest-and-digest state.

Unfortunately, our modern-day sabre tooth tiger neither roars nor bites. It looks more like this.

- Caring for aging parents
- Financial stress
- Late for work again
- Marital problems
- Not enough time in a day to get everything done
- Overbearing boss
- Stuck in traffic
- Unruly children

When faced with stress, you experience the same physiological response as your primitive ancestor. Unlike her, you are stuck in a cubicle at work, in your car or inside your house. You have no one to fight and nowhere to flee. All the energy released by cortisol remains unused, causing weight gain, especially in the abdomen; this makes you more susceptible to obesity and diabetes. The huge release of adrenaline also remains unused, raising your risk for heart disease and high blood pressure.

Because you don't experience the same physical release in your stressful situations, you will find it more difficult to return to a state of calm and balance. Without that release, the stress response fails to shut off after a difficult event has passed. Therefore you remain in a fight-or-flight state, which perpetuates the cycle of stress.

Later in this chapter, you will learn healthy ways to help you cope with stress and successfully come back to a state of rest-and-digest.

> " Underlying every serious malady that
> you can think of is chronic stress. "
> —Alexander Dhand

Though you may not be running away from a sabre tooth tiger, the stress you face today is adversely affecting your well-being. If you neglect to find ways to deal with it, prolonged stress will cause damage to your health.

In 1936, Hans Selye coined the term *stress*. He observed that laboratory animals subjected to distressing physical and emotional stimuli showed physical changes. The animals were exposed to extremes of heat and cold, blaring light, deafening sound and perpetual frustration. The changes noted were an enlargement of the adrenals, shrinkage of the lymph tissue and stomach ulcerations. He later demonstrated that persistent exposure to stress in these animals caused them to develop diseases similar to those in humans, such as heart attacks, stroke, kidney disease and rheumatoid arthritis.

I recently spoke with Alexander Dhand, a registered psychologist at Momentum Health. He repeatedly emphasized the seriousness of stress.

> I'm an evangelist for trying to convince people to take stress seriously. The main issue with stress is chronic stress. That is very much a feature of our lives. For example, both partners working outside the home, looking after the home front and the children. This all leads to chronic stress as the main issue.

More and more women over 40 are taking centre stage in the business community and are expected to perform well in and out of the home. In addition to their day jobs, they still face the challenge of balancing their schedules in order to accommodate children, spouses, parents, relatives and friends. A career woman is present at her children's school and sporting activities, deals with domestic chores and attends to the shopping, as well as many other errands. She is sometimes so busy taking care of everyone else that she forgets about herself, resulting in poor nutrition, lack of sleep, no exercise and no time to spend on herself. Is this sounding familiar?

Mr. Dhand continues.

> What makes chronic stress a real issue from the standpoint of health is that stress is directly related to the suppression of the immune system. People who are chronically stressed are much more susceptible to things like catching a cold or flu, or to the nastier things like cancers of various sorts. The body's ability to defend itself is reduced. Underlying every serious malady that you can think of is chronic stress. It is said that depression is fast approaching the number one health problem globally. But I would say it's not depression—it's actually stress. Chronic stress is the number one health problem globally.

Health Problems Related to Chronic Stress

Chronic stress can cause a cascading series of physiological responses in your body that may lead to serious health issues such as these.

- **Adrenal fatigue:** The adrenal glands are responsible for producing the stress hormones cortisol and adrenaline, and so prolonged stress can exhaust them, leaving you feeling overwhelmed, depressed and prone to chronic fatigue.

- **Cancer:** Because stress decreases the body's ability to fight disease, it loses the ability to kill cancer cells.

- **Cardiovascular disease:** Increased LDL (the "bad" cholesterol), triglycerides and blood pressure, and the aggregation of blood platelets, increase your risk of developing cardiovascular diseases. According to the World Health Organization's 2014 global status report on noncommunicable diseases, cardiovascular diseases are the number one cause of death globally. More people die annually from cardiovascular diseases than from any other cause.

- **Depression:** Chronically elevated levels of cortisol can cause low serotonin levels resulting in depression. If left unchecked, this common disorder can lead to more serious mental illness.

- **Diabetes:** Chronic stress can significantly increase a person's risk of developing type 2 diabetes because the body becomes insulin resistant, leading to high blood sugar.

- **Imbalance of female hormones:** Prolonged stress leads to an imbalance of the female hormones, estrogen and progesterone. This causes unpleasant physical and emotional problems such as hot flashes, depression, irritability and chronic fatigue.

- **Obesity:** When the body reacts to chronic stress, the cortisol hormone is secreted in higher quantities. Cortisol mobilizes blood glucose for energy. This unused extra energy is deposited as fat that is stored deep in the abdomen.

 Stress can also lead to a craving for comfort foods such as sugary treats and other simple carbohydrates. These signal the brain to produce serotonin, which has a temporary calming effect on the mind and body. We repeatedly eat these comfort foods in an effort to calm ourselves in times of stress, which leads to extra weight.

- **Osteoporosis:** Elevated levels of cortisol in times of stress cause calcium depletion of bone tissue. This can reduce bone density, which may lead to osteoporosis.

Fourteen Ways to Help You Relax

Stress in small doses can be beneficial for us in terms of increased energy and alertness while completing an important task. This type of stress is considered good. But when life becomes overwhelming, it is important to learn how to slow things down. Relaxation is a key component in stress relief.

Applying relaxation techniques can help reduce stress symptoms by slowing your heart and breathing rate, lowering your blood pressure, and reducing your muscular tension. This results in the stress hormones returning to normal levels.

Being able to relax results in:

- Better sleep
- Decreased muscular pain
- Improved breathing
- Improved concentration
- Improved digestion
- Improved immunity
- Reduced fatigue

Relaxation can be as simple as playing your favourite music, having a bath or getting a massage. Through relaxation, you can achieve a positive response to stress and its associated symptoms and disorders. Find ways to make relaxation a part of your daily routine. Take time out to give your body and mind a much needed break.

Here are some tools and activities you can incorporate into your daily or weekly routine to help you experience relaxation and relief from stress and its symptoms. With stress being the culprit associated with many modern-day diseases, these simple ideas can be effective ways to help you manage and overcome stress and its harmful effects.

1. Meditation, Deep Breathing and Yoga

Meditation takes you deeper into yourself;
it's getting to know your inner person.
—Ann Dowling

Meditation and deep breathing are practices associated with the tradition of yoga. They can help your mind and body return to a place of peace. It may seem simple, but the rhythmic pattern of breath in and breath out has a very calming and soothing quality.

While following this quiet rhythm, your breathing rate slows down, which in turn relaxes your entire body. With each deep breath in, your diaphragm is drawn downwards towards the liver, stomach and other organs. When exhaling, your diaphragm then moves upwards towards the heart. That creates an internal massage of these tissues, which detoxifies them and improves blood and lymph flow. This boosts the immune system, and reduces stress and fatigue. The deeper the breath, the more oxygen is taken in helping your body to release endorphins—the feel-good hormones. This has a relaxing and re-energizing effect on your mind and body, leaving you with a greater sense of well-being. Find 10–15 minutes to be alone with your breath.

My dear friend Ann Dowling was very open about sharing her story. Listen as she explains how chronic stress left her vulnerable to the effects of cancer.

> In December of 2010, when I was in my late 50s, I went for a routine mammogram. When the technician said that they needed to redo one of my mammograms, I felt this little wave of panic. They didn't allude to anything. They just said that the doctor would be in touch with me. After two seemingly long days, I got a call from the doctor requesting to see me in his office to discuss one of my tests. A week later, I had a biopsy done, and at that point, I was diagnosed with breast cancer. Hearing this was a shock! Although I had many friends who had been diagnosed with cancer, you never think it's going to be you.

Ann is a busy executive assistant with a major airline. I asked her if she thought that what happened to her was directly related to the stress in her life.

Definitely! These were very busy times. With the children gone away to university, I was assuming extra work. You tend to fill that void with more work and longer hours. It was my way of trying not to miss them too much. I was trying to incorporate exercise into my day. But waking up at 4:00 a.m. to get my workout in was adding to the stress. I had no balance. Then my mom passed away. I found myself trying to deal with that too. Longer hours at work, Mom's passing, kids gone—I would definitely say that stress was related to it. The stress was not just in those few months; it was years of it.

When you're going through this, it seems so unbelievable. Is this really happening to me? I kept my diagnosis to myself for a couple of weeks because my husband was in China on business, and my children were busy with finals. I did not want to hit them with this news, especially because I did not know all the facts at this point. I didn't even want to tell my own sisters because I needed to share this with my husband first. Keeping this information to myself was also quite stressful! My husband scolded me a little for not having told him sooner. My children were also definitely worried when they came home for Christmas.

I finally had the surgery followed by radiation. All went well. After the surgery, they held a seminar for the patients. They talked about a variety of great classes they had to offer. One of them was an eight-week meditation course. I had heard of meditation but had never actively pursued it. I was very open to it; it seemed like the right path to follow. I was ready for some healing.

A nurse at the hospital gave the meditation course. It was a very small group. I really enjoyed our sessions, and there were many feelings shared. It was wonderful!

I asked Ann to share with me the many benefits she experienced from practicing meditation. Here are the four most important things she told me.

1. Joy

   After my eight-week meditation course, I joined a yoga class for cancer survivors. Our instructor, Claudia, would take us into meditation at the end of yoga practice. It was just as they say: the sun, the moon, and the stars aligned. I think meditation takes you deeper into yourself; it's getting to know your inner person. I was filled with a sense of well-being. I felt an inner happiness, a joy.

2. Priorities

   Meditation also helped me start to put things into proper perspective. For example, do I really need to do that right now? Not everything has to have a now place. I incorporated this new outlook at home as well as at work. Before, all the tasks that were in front of me were to be done today! Now, I prioritize. If it's something that's important to me, it gets done first.

3. Time for Me

   Saturday is typically the day I do household chores. But I don't spend my whole day cleaning the house now. I put myself first and take time for me. It can be something like reading a book. I'm not going to feel guilty about it. It's for me, and it's for my well-being!

4. Inner Balance

   I also began to feel a sense of inner balance. When that inner balance is achieved, it also expresses itself on the outside. People see it. I have had people tell me I look different, younger! Now, five years later, I am happy to say that I am not on any medication, and I am cancer-free!

Congratulations to Ann for being cancer-free and for having developed a deeper appreciation for herself and the importance of her well-being.

Ann's yoga instructor, Claudia, explained that there is much evidence-based research showing how the tools of yoga can help you manage stress. Yoga is being used for people who are dealing with post-traumatic stress disorder, people who have chronic health conditions and people who are living with day-to-day stress in their lives.

> In yoga philosophy, our being is thought of as an onion. There are these layers upon layers; they are called the koshas. There is the physical body, the breath body, the emotional body and the cognitive body, then there is this layer of joy or bliss. When you're looking at stress relief, you might be touching into that emotional body and perhaps clearing away deeply-held emotions that are lodged in your body. You begin to release this. In that way you create more ease in your being.

> At the end of the class, you lie in a Savasana, a corpse pose. You see people experience this sense of well-being or joy. Yoga practice allows us to move through these other fluctuating layers to touch into these deeper aspects of ourselves. In so doing, we come to touch this layer of joy, which is an expression of our true nature, our true selves—the centre of our being.

Meditation for Beginners

The well-documented benefits of meditation are as follows.

- A feeling of vitality and rejuvenation
- Better learning ability
- Decreased depression
- Greater creativity
- Improved memory
- Less anxiety
- Less stress

- Lower blood pressure
- Reduction in irritability and moodiness

While studying to become a yoga instructor, Tania Hernandez discovered the value of meditation and how regular practice helps you achieve an overall sense of peace and well-being.

> I finally understood the critical importance of meditation, and how it is an effective way to release stress. If we were to take about 10 minutes every single day to meditate, we would give ourselves the opportunity to experience an internal peace that is released by self-love.

> We nourish our physical body all the time with food and sleep. However, our minds are always racing a million miles per second. We must take care of that. We can do so by releasing built-up tension and stress through exercise, and by quieting our minds through meditation.

> I truly believe that meditation can help in the most important area of your life, your inner self. Taking care of that allows you to treat your outer body with much more love and respect. You will naturally want to exercise, eat healthier and embrace this gift called life.

Deep Breathing

Here is a simple deep breathing technique that will help place you in a peaceful, meditative state.

- Lie or sit comfortably. Your entire posture should be relaxed, with no feeling of strain on any part of your body.
- Close your eyes to avoid external distractions.
- Place your hands on your abdomen.
- Relax your shoulders.

- Take slow, deep breaths in and out through your nose. Allow your breathing to fall into a comfortable pattern, and pay attention to it as it passes in and out of your nose.
- Concentrate on the rhythmic movement of the abdomen rising as you breathe in and falling as you breathe out.

  Repeat a word or phrase to help you focus. The phrase I use is, "Breathe in [as I inhale] and let it go [as I exhale]."

  "Breathe in and let it go!"

- Let go of your thoughts. If you find your thoughts wandering, try naming the distractions as a way of setting them aside. For example, say in your mind, "Worried about work," then gently bring yourself back to your breathing.

  Continue for 5–10 minutes, then open your eyes and sit or lie there for a moment.

Deep breathing and meditation can calm your body and mind, leaving you revitalized, refreshed and energized.

Yoga for Beginners

If you are new to yoga, the child's pose (Balasana) is a great beginning yoga pose. It is very beneficial during times of stress. It calms the central nervous system, leaving you with a greater sense of physical and mental relief. Take a moment to practice the child's pose.

Child's Pose (Balasana)

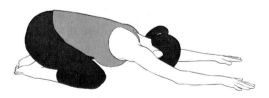

- Begin on your knees. Choose a soft surface (yoga mat, blanket, or towel).
- Keep your big toes touching and spread your knees.

- Exhale and lower your torso until your belly touches your thighs and your forehead rests on the mat. If you cannot reach all the way down, rest your forehead on a rolled-up towel.
- Place your arms along your sides, or extend them overhead.
- Focus on pressing your hips into your heels. Don't worry if you cannot do this in the beginning. With practice, you will be able to rest your hips comfortably on your heels.
- Keep breathing in and out to increase the stretch and relaxation.
- Hold the pose for 20 seconds to one minute.

As you have learned, breathing is an important part of relaxation. Focus on your breathing while in child's pose. With each breath in, feel your spine lengthening and your torso expanding. As you exhale, let go of your tension and immerse yourself deeper into relaxation.

2. Massage Therapy

" Massage is something I do for myself,
something I look forward to. "
—Shannon

Massage therapy is commonly used for pain relief and relaxation. By manipulating the soft tissues, a trained massage therapist can assist your muscles to return to their natural, relaxed state. When physical tension is reduced, mental tension also melts away. In addition, research has shown that massage can lower your heart rate and blood pressure, adding to the relaxation effect. It also increases the production of endorphins, which helps to boost your mood.

Shannon, a 48-year-old social worker, explains how massage therapy helps her manage her stress levels resulting in better pain management for her fibromyalgia.

I believe that fibromyalgia is a physical issue because it manifests in pain. Its control, however, is stress management to some degree. Some people might disagree with me. There are many times where my pain acts up, and I have no idea what set it off. When I keep a pain journal, I find that pain peaks five days after a stressor.

I know that without sleep, exercise, proper nutrition or stress management techniques, I would live in a state of constant chronic pain. Just like diabetes, heart disease and multiple sclerosis, fibromyalgia is also exacerbated by stress.

Massage is one of the techniques I use for stress management. It helps release the pain and keeps me going. It's also something I do for myself, something I look forward to. As a social worker, I remind my clients, especially those struggling with depression, to have something to look forward to.

There are so many reasons why you should visit your massage therapist regularly, especially during times of stress. Find a qualified therapist near you, and begin to enjoy the incredible benefits that come from consistent treatments.

3. Stretching

Stretching is very closely related to yoga. It can serve as relaxation and rejuvenation for the mind and body—a great tool to help relieve tension. Taking time to stretch can help you slow down and refocus your energy. Forward bends, whether seated or standing, are very soothing for the nervous system. See chapter 4, which includes an illustrated stretching routine.

4. Exercise

Regular physical activity is a healthy way to relieve tension and help you manage stress. Exercise stimulates the production of endorphins, which has a positive effect on your emotional state. Walking, running, gardening, dancing—even just 20 minutes of continuous exercise can have great benefits for your body and mind.

Something as simple as a daily walk can be a powerful relaxation technique. It is easy to do and is available to all. Take your worries outdoors, find a pretty place and walk a while. It is a constructive method of releasing physical energy and emotional stress. It will help get your mind off your concerns and daily pressures. Look for simple ways to increase your daily physical activity. See chapter 4, which includes an illustrated workout routine.

5. Reconnect with Nature

> " I go to nature to be soothed and healed,
> and to have my senses put in order. "
> —John Burroughs

I was on my cell phone one day trying to get online, but all I got was a grey screen. My phone was on the blink! My first instinct was to text one of my sons and ask him what I should do. Then I remembered something he told me the last time I had an issue: "Mom, just turn it off, let it sit for a while and then turn it on again, and everything will work better!" That's exactly what I did. He was right, and I was back online in no time.

A week later, I was feeling much like my phone. I too was on the blink. I needed some time away from life to "turn it off" and recharge. I decided to pack food, water and a few warm jackets, and then I set off for the mountains.

The long drive through the beautiful mountains was so invigorating. I stopped along the way to have a solo picnic by the river, and then I continued on to my destination, an emerald lake nestled in the majestic Rocky Mountains. It was paradise! The view was so breathtaking that it instantly soothed my soul. The peaceful lake with its backdrop of snow-capped mountains was just what I needed. I picked a spot by the lake and sat for a while, taking in this glorious sight. I continued my day with a long hike up the side of the mountain, catching glimpses of the magnificent lake below through the pine forest. This experience filled me with a wonderful healing energy—something only nature can provide.

It is good to occasionally reconnect with nature and be alone with your thoughts without being surrounded by the noise of daily life. You will feel recharged, feel reenergized, and able to function better in life. This will allow you to give your best and be at your best. Your body and your mind will feel refreshed and ready to take on daily challenges with renewed energy and passion.

6. Aromatherapy

Essential oils can help relieve stress. Specific scents are used to induce feelings of relaxation. Chamomile, citrus, eucalyptus, lavender, rose, and vanilla are just a few of the scents used to promote a sense of calm and serenity.

The most popular of all essential oils is lavender. Just a few drops of this sweet floral scent can be an effective and pleasant way to help you experience relaxation both physically and emotionally.

Here are some ways to apply a few drops of lavender.

- Blend with a carrier oil such as almond oil, and massage into skin
- In a bath
- In a diffuser
- In a mist bottle (10 drops to 100 mL water); spray on your hair, on your face with eyes closed or in a room
- On a warm compress
- On the back of your neck
- On the soles of your feet
- On your pillow before going to bed

7. Tea

Any hot, caffeine-free tea may be relaxing. Chamomile and lemon balm are nervine herbs that are especially soothing to the nervous system. A cup of chamomile or lemon balm tea before bed will encourage a sense of calm and relaxation and promote restful sleep. Try a cup tonight!

8. Rescue Remedy (Bach Flower Remedy)

Rescue Remedy is a homeopathic blend of five flowers, discovered by Dr. Edward Bach in the early 1900s. Place five drops under your tongue during stressful situations to help you feel relaxed, calm and focused. It is also great when taken at bedtime, if you are feeling restless. It is commonly available at your local health food store.

9. Gratitude Journal and Prayer

Stress can conjure up all kinds of negative emotions. Have a journal handy and record things for which you are grateful. You can also try pouring out your gratitude in prayer. Focusing on all the positive things in your life during stressful times can shift your attention away from the stressor.

10. Relaxing Music

Play your favourite relaxation music at the office, in the car, in the bath or wherever you need it most. Soothing music is a great remedy for stress. It has a way of calming the nerves, slowing the heart rate and lowering levels of cortisol.

11. Magnesium

Magnesium serves to reduce the nerve excitation caused by stress. Great dietary sources of magnesium are:

- Beans and lentils
- Brown rice

- Leafy green vegetables
- Pumpkin seeds and brazil nuts
- Salmon and mackerel

A supplement may also be beneficial. Check with your doctor.

12. Sleep

Getting enough sleep allows you to perform at your best. Ideally, seven to eight hours of sleep a night is recommended. Your body needs that time to regenerate both physically and mentally. With adequate rest, you will be better prepared to meet the day's challenges. Pushing yourself too hard on too little sleep will eventually wear you out, leaving you vulnerable to many stress-related health problems. See chapter 6 for tips to help you improve sleep.

13. Epsom Salts Bath

Epsom salts are magnesium sulphate mineral salts. Magnesium sulphate in a hot bath encourages relaxation. The warm, soothing atmosphere of having a bath sends an immediate message to your mind that it is time to relax. This is a perfect way to unwind at the end of the day.

- Fill a bathtub with water as hot as is comfortable.
- Add one to two cups of Epsom salts crystals to your bath water; stir and allow this to dissolve.
- Add a few drops of essential oils to your bath water to increase the relaxation effect. Lavender is an excellent choice.

You may also choose to play relaxing music and light a few candles to help you unwind.

An Epsom salts bath can be a great addition to your stress-reduction regimen. You will be assured of a great night's sleep that will help regenerate and revitalize you.

Epsom salts may not be recommended for those suffering from high blood pressure, a heart condition or diabetes. Check with your doctor.

14. Talk to a Friend

Having a close friend or a loved one you can talk to can certainly help relieve the burdens of stress. It should be someone trustworthy—one who will listen, support you and provide positive feedback. Talking can be a great release of emotions. Sometimes the simple act of talking can also help you find a solution to the problem that might be causing you stress. Call a friend today!

With regular application of one or more of these suggestions for relaxation, you will be better equipped to deal with the stress in your life. Was there one suggestion that resonated with you? Begin implementing it today and experience for yourself the sweet feeling of relaxation and the release of stressful emotions.

Food and Stress

Stress can have a negative effect on your overall health. Are you getting the nutrients your body needs to stay healthy? Here are some basic principles of good nutrition.

- Begin your day with a good breakfast.
- Continue your day by making healthy food choices. Ensure you include protein, carbohydrates and healthy fats at every meal.
- Build your diet around fresh vegetables and fruit, beans and lentils, whole grains, nuts and seeds, and lean meat.
- Eat smaller meals at regular intervals (every three to four hours) to give your body a constant flow of nutrients.
- Drink at least eight glasses of water a day.
- Ensure that you have an adequate intake of vitamins and minerals.

Here are some additional dietary guidelines that will help you in times of stress.

Foods That Help Reduce Stress

- **Complex carbohydrates:** Complex carbohydrates such as whole grains, starchy vegetables, and beans and lentils help to stabilize blood sugar levels and prompt the release of serotonin, which has a calming effect.

- **Vitamin C:** Fruits such as berries and citrus fruits help strengthen the immune system, which can be compromised by stress.

- **Magnesium:** Magnesium is depleted in response to stress. Eat more green leafy vegetables, which are especially high in magnesium. They are also high in the B vitamins to help support healthy mood.

- **Omega-3 fatty acids:** Fatty acids found in foods such as salmon, flax seed oil, chia seeds and walnuts help prevent surges of the stress hormones.

- **Potassium:** Foods high in potassium such as bananas, dark leafy greens and squash help to balance the nervous system and calm anxiety.

- **Protein:** Including protein at every meal will stabilize your blood sugar levels. This will help curb your hunger so you will not turn to traditional comfort foods, which can exacerbate stress. Good protein choices are chicken and fish, eggs, plain yogurt, beans and lentils, and nuts and seeds.

- **Water:** Dehydration can occur during stressful times because the heart rate is raised and you are breathing harder. This state of dehydration can lead to an increase in cortisol. The recommended daily intake is at least eight glasses of purified water.

Foods That Aggravate Stress

- **Alcohol:** The body's response to alcohol is similar to the stress response. Most people reach for alcohol to help calm them down, but the opposite is true. Alcohol stimulates the production of cortisol, the same hormone produced in times of stress.

- **Caffeine:** Whether it be coffee, caffeinated tea or energy drinks, caffeine intensifies stress by stimulating the adrenal glands to release cortisol. In addition, many caffeinated drinks are loaded with sugar; this also raises cortisol levels.

- **Processed food:** This type of food usually contains sugar, salt, fat, chemicals and artificial ingredients with little nutritional value to help sustain you in times of stress. Processed foods are also high in calories, which can lead to weight gain. This increases psychological stress. Some examples of processed foods are frozen dinners, bagged salty snacks, store-bought baked goods, sugary cereals and deli meats.

- **Sugary treats:** With increased dietary sugar, blood glucose levels spike. This raises levels of cortisol. Some sugary treats to avoid are candy, chocolate bars, soft drinks, store-bought fruit juice and cookies.

By eating a nutritious and balanced diet, you will be better equipped to deal with stress and repair the damage caused by it.

Learn to Prioritize

> For me, that's what stress is about: you're just not prioritizing.
> —Lana Dunn

Most women over 40 are busy juggling the demands of a job, family, chores and other commitments. It sometimes seems like there are not enough hours in a day. You may feel constantly under pressure to fulfil all these roles, and this can leave you vulnerable to stress. You can ease the burden of stress by applying proper time management techniques to your daily schedule. This ensures that the time available will be used more efficiently.

The first step is to evaluate how you are spending your time, looking for sections of time that can be used more wisely. The next thing is to prioritize, which ensures that your time and energy are spent on truly important tasks.

Lana Dunn is a psychologist with Heroic Living. She feels that most health problems of today, such as anxiety and depression, are related to lifestyle and stress. She often encourages her clients to use their time more wisely and to prioritize in order to minimize their stress levels.

> I feel that people are too quick to start on medication, which becomes a bigger continual problem. They are always ready for a quick fix as opposed to making some lifestyle changes. I always get my clients to first start looking at what they are drinking and eating. I believe that you cannot feel calm if you are constantly filling your body with junk.

> The next thing I have them do is track their activity over a couple of days to start identifying how much time they spend on certain things. People often say, "I have no time," "I feel rushed," and "I'm so busy." This exercise gives them a sense of just how they spend their day and their hours.

> I also have them do a really simple four-by-four grid. One quadrant is for necessary activities, and one quadrant is for unnecessary ones. One quadrant is for important activities, and one quadrant is for unimportant ones.

I have my clients look at what things fall within the quadrants of necessary and important. They should be focusing most of their attention on those things.

Next, I encourage them to examine the things that fall under the unnecessary yet important quadrant. These can be things such as watching a TV show with their spouse every night.

Then I have my clients really look at what things land in that unnecessary and unimportant place, and how to stop spending time on that. This is where people might realize that, for example, they spent two hours on Facebook yesterday.

Some people think that they are not responsible for their stress. Once they realize that it is how they choose to spend their time that is causing them stress, they begin to regain control. That's really the biggest thing—to invite people to that awareness. For me, that's what stress is about: you're just not prioritizing. It is about being able to do that for yourself.

Similar to Lana's method, Steven R. Covey created a system to better organize your activities by classifying them into four categories. This approach, explained below in chart form, will help you prioritize, reducing stress.

	Urgent	Not Urgent
Important	I Activities: • Crises • Pressing problems • Deadline-driven projects	II Activities: • Relationship building • Planning, goal setting • Recreation, exercising
Not Important	III Activities: • Interruptions • Unnecessary meetings • Proximate, pressing matters	IV Activities: • Trivia, busy work • Time wasters • Pleasant activities

Adapted from Stephen R. Covey's book
The 7 Habits of Highly Effective People

Here are some examples of things that might fall into each of the four quadrants.

	Urgent	Not Urgent
Important	I Activities: • Car breaks down • Personal injury • Project deadline looming	II Activities: • Family time • Relaxing, reading • Creating meal plans • Going to the gym
Not Important	III Activities: • Responding to every text, phone call or e-mail • Child's trivial demands • House always as neat as a pin	IV Activities: • Watching TV • Checking Facebook • Browsing social media

Quadrant I: Important, Urgent

All of these activities require immediate action, and some have an important deadline. You must meet your commitments and deal with crises as they arise. But having too many of these activities in your life will increase your stress, make you feel like you have lost control and eventually lead to frustration and fatigue.

Advice: Review your list and prioritize the activities. Are they all truly important and urgent? Do those activities that are the most urgent first. Perhaps you can enlist the help of a friend or family member to assist you in accomplishing these things.

In the future, try to anticipate things and work ahead so that important activities do not become urgent.

Quadrant II: Important, Not Urgent

Because these activities are not urgent, you may need to schedule them and then stick to your schedule. These activities are important because they help you reduce your stress and improve your overall performance. They can prevent crises from developing and give you a sense of fulfilment. Unfortunately, we sometimes mistake the more urgent activities as being important, and we push back these activities for later. Occasionally they don't get done at all, leading us back to a place of stress.

Advice: Ideally, this quadrant is where you should be spending most of your time. Schedule a time at the beginning of the week to make your list of the things that are important to you but may not be urgent. Check your list each evening to make sure you are accomplishing the things you set out to do.

Quadrant III: Not Important, Urgent

These activities often come upon you unexpectedly. Because they are urgent, they steal your attention. Sometimes these come as a request to cater to someone else's urgency. Be aware that you can say no, or "not at this moment." These urgent-but-not-important demands can disrupt your plans, leaving you less time and energy for the really important things.

Advice: Many of these you can ignore or do later, after the important things are done. They may not be as urgent as you might first believe. Remember to be polite, but don't automatically accept everyone else's requests for your time.

Quadrant IV: Not Important, Not Urgent

These activities are wasteful distractions. Doing these activities may seem like they are helping you reduce your stress, when in fact you are falling further behind on things you should be doing. And eventually, when deadlines catch up with you, you will feel even more stressed because you have wasted time and accomplished nothing.

Advice: Limit these activities or eliminate them altogether. Make it part of your plan to avoid spending time and energy on these things.

From my own personal experience, using the four-quadrant method has helped me achieve my goal of finishing the manuscript for *Healthy Body for Life*. This is something that I really wanted to accomplish, and therefore I gave it top priority. I let people around me know about my goal, and they were very good about not taking up my time with their to-do lists. In addition, reading and responding to e-mails no longer took place first thing in the morning. I used this time of day, when I felt more energized and creative, to write my book. E-mails could wait until later.

I took the time to do the things that were important but not necessarily urgent. Saturday was still date night, and Sundays were still a time for spiritual things and for family dinners. Balance helped me feel less stressed and made it easier for me to focus on the task at hand.

I also spent little time in the not-important, not-urgent category. It would have been easy for me to watch television or spend time on social media.

I am happy to say that by making the conscious choice of not having the unimportant things rob me of my time, I can now present you with my finished book, *Healthy Body for Life—A Guide for Women over 40*!

I invite you to use this blank form to list the activities that have occupied your time this past week. This exercise will help you become more aware of where you are spending your time and how you are currently prioritizing. In order to reduce your stress, I encourage you to commit to making changes that will free up more time for the important things in your life which are not of an urgent nature. These will lead to less stress and more success.

	Urgent	Not Urgent
Important	I	II
Not Important	III	IV

Now that you have learned to establish your priorities, the next step is to schedule your activities. You can use a schedule similar to the one below, or you can use a calendar, an appointment book, a spreadsheet, or a phone app. Find a system that works best for you. Remember the importance of scheduling time for yourself, your family and your friends so that you can experience a more balanced life.

Times	Weekly	Schedule					
	Monday	Tuesday	Wednesday	Thursday	Friday	Saturday	Sunday
6:00							
7:00							
8:00							
9:00							
10:00							
11:00							
12:00							
PM							
1:00							
2:00							
3:00							
4:00							
5:00							
6:00							
7:00							
8:00							
9:00							
10:00							

“ Our culture encourages us to plan every moment
and fill our schedules with one activity and
obligation after the next, with no time to just be.
But the human body and mind require downtime
to rejuvenate. I have found my greatest moments
of joy and peace just sitting in silence, and then I
take that joy and peace with me out into the world. ”
—Holly Mosier

A FINAL WORD

Ready for Change

> " You are never too young to learn,
> never too old to change. "
> —Thomas S. Monson

Thank you for taking this journey with me. After reading *Healthy Body for Life*, ask yourself this question: "How am I going to live differently from this day forward?"

The pathway to wellness for women over 40 need not be complicated or overwhelming. I encourage you to put into practice what you have learned by introducing small changes into your life. Are there some changes you have already made as a result of the chapters you have read? What difference has this made in your life?

It is my sincerest wish that *Healthy Body for Life* has inspired you to make a change. I hope you feel motivated to continue to adopt the tools I have shared with you. Discover for yourself what it means to live a healthier, happier life in your 40s and well beyond.

Embrace this time of your life. Take care of yourself both physically and mentally, and move forward with a positive outlook.

I leave you with my personal mission statement and my encouragement.

Eat well, stay active, live happy!